Spintronics

Spintronics

Spirituality, Mental Health and Quality of Life

Naveen Pant

Spirituality, Mental Health and Quality of Life

Pathways in Indian Psychology

Springer

Naveen Pant
Department of Psychology
Gurukula Kangri (Deemed to be University)
Haridwar, Uttarakhand, India

ISBN 978-981-99-2702-9 ISBN 978-981-99-2703-6 (eBook)
https://doi.org/10.1007/978-981-99-2703-6

This Springer imprint is published by the registered company Springer Nature Singapore Pte Ltd.
The registered company address is: 152 Beach Road, #21-01/04 Gateway East, Singapore 189721, Singapore

Dedicated to my Mata ji,
Shree Ist-Kul Dev Shiva and Pandav Vansi Maharaaj,
Great Grandfather Shree Lal Pant Vedya, and
Grandfather

About This Book

Spirituality is the core concept of transpersonal psychology, and mental health has been a focal point of studies, research and talks from the starting point of psychology and earlier health and wellbeing sciences. So, encompassing all the concepts of spirituality, mental health, quality of life and Indian psychology in a single book requires a hybrid approach. Research and exploration of the relations between Indian psychology and modern psychology is a major part of the book. Mental health and related problems are increasing rapidly, and this is a matter of concern, yet there is not even a unanimous and empirical approach to assess and cure it, due to its diversity and other causes. This book is based on the most developed construct: spiritual intelligence and aims to discover its effects on mental health and quality of life. Spirituality and its other constructs are one of the most interesting topics nowadays in the area of positive/indigenous/transpersonal psychology and among social and behavioural scientists. This book provides material on spirituality, spiritual intelligence, mental health and quality of life. It then attempts to review related literature, both review and empirical, and to explore past and current scenarios on spirituality and mental health and quality of life research. The fourth chapter of the book is the author's original empirical research report on 'The role of spirituality in predicting mental health and quality of life among early adults'. The fifth chapter provides a look at mental health and the mind from an Indian psychological perspective, proposing an 'Indian model of personality'. Finally, in the sixth chapter, the book has a thorough look at Indian psychology in view of modern psychological concepts. In summary, Chapters 1 and 2 present material on spirituality, mental health and quality of life; Chapters 3 and 4 contain the review and empirical research done by the author in the said area; and Chapters 5 and 6 contain information on Indian psychology and explore modern psychological concepts found in Indian indigenous texts, such as: the Bhagvad Gita, Yoga, Veda, Atharva Veda, Ayurveda, Upanishads, Jyotisha, Vastu Shastra, Samudrik Shastra, Kaam Shastra and the legacies of Indian scholars. This book will provide the stuff of current demand for hybrid research and a new look at the emerging fields, which will be a special focus of interest among students, teachers, researchers, mental health professionals, quality of life scholars, Indian psychologists, and indigenous psychologists.

Contents

About the Author

Dr. Naveen Pant is currently working as an assistant professor in the Department of Psychology, Gurukula Kangri (Deemed to be University), Haridwar, India. Prior to this Dr Pant has worked as an academic counsellor (Psychology), at UOU Study Centre, MBGPG College, Haldwani, India. Dr. Pant has contributed more than 13 international and national research papers, has worked as a member of editorial and reviewer boards in more than four reputed journals, contributed two book chapters. Dr. Pant has more than ten years of academic and research experience in the field. His areas of expertise and interest are indigenous/Indian psychology and mental health. He was also awarded the 'Young Scientist Award' (2020, Hyderabad, India).

Abbreviations

CBT	Cognitive Behavioural Therapy
EQ	Emotional Intelligence (Quotient)
HRQOL	Health-related Quality of Life
IQ	Intelligence Quotient
ISIS	Integrated Spiritual Intelligence Scale
MH	Mental Health
MMHSI	Mithila Mental Health Status Inventory
NPC	Normal Probability Curve
PQ	Physical Intelligence (Quotient)
QoL	Quality of life
SD	Standard Deviation
SI	Spiritual Intelligence
SQ	Spiritual Intelligence (Quotient)
WHOQOL-100	World Health Organization Quality of Life Scale (Long Version)
WHOQOL-BREF	WHO Quality of Life-Brief (Short Version Scale)

Key English Transliterated (Hindi/Sanskrit) Words

Serial No.	English Transliteration	Hindi/ Sanskrit Words
1.	Bhagvad Gita	भगवद्गीता
2.	Shree Krishna	श्री कृष्ण
3.	Upanishad	उपनिषद्
4.	Yoga	योग
5.	Mahabharata	महाभारत
6.	Veda	वेद
7.	Ayurveda	आयुर्वेद
8.	Vedanta	वेदांत
9.	Maharishi Charaka	महर्षि चरक
10.	Maharishi Shushruta	महर्षि शुश्रुत

Serial No.	English Transliteration	Hindi/ Sanskrit Words
11.	Prakruti (Nature): Saatvik, Rajsik, Taamsik	प्रकृति- सात्विक, राजसिक, तामसिक
12.	Tri Guna: Sattva, Rajas, Tamas	त्रिगुण- सत्व, रजस, तमस
13.	Tri Doshas: Vata, Pitta, Kapha	त्रिदोष- वात, पित्त, कफ
14.	Tri Yogas: Karma, Bhakti, Gyan	त्रियोग- कर्म, भक्ति, ज्ञान
15.	Dharma	धर्म
16.	Pancha Koshas (Five Sheaths)	पंच कोश
17.	Jeeva	जीव
18.	Manas, Man (Mind)	मनस, मन
19.	Buddhi (Intellect)	बुद्धि
20.	Ahankara	अहंकार
21.	Kaam Shastra	कामशास्त्र
22.	Chetna (Consciousness)	चेतना
23.	Shareer (Body): Sthool, Sooksma, Karan	शरीर- स्थूल, सूक्ष्म, कारण
24.	Pragyaaparadha (Intellectual Error)	प्रज्ञापराध
25.	Jyotisha, Vastu, Shamudrik Shastra	ज्योतिष, वास्तु, सामुद्रिक शास्त्र

List of Figures

List of Tables

Chapter 1
Introduction

Spirituality is the core concept of Transpersonal Psychology, and mental health has been a focal point of the study, research, and talks from the earliest starting point of Psychology and past health and wellbeing sciences. For getting a quick seem of the entire book in a single chapter, this first chapter is formulated as. This chapter explores the concept of spirituality, religiosity, mental health, and quality of life and examines the relationship among the above-said concepts. Researchers and clinicians observed that improvement of spiritual and religious qualities; values and resources affect health and intervention. The chapter also reviews past studies related to these concepts. Finally, this chapter suggests some alleviating notions of mental as well as physical health which are part of Indian Psychological perspectives. Findings of past researches indicate that spirituality and religiosity have a significant and strong relationship with both mental health and quality of life. And there is enough stuff about health and mental health in Indian Psychology to cure it authentically.

1.1 Spirituality

Spirituality has specific implications from diverse perspectives. Spirituality in lay usage means something related to religiosity and the religion of the community. Spirituality in common sense may be related to God or be immaterial; from a psychological point of view it is an ultimate intelligence, and in Indian psychology (philosophy) it is a way of life to find the ultimate truth. The adjectival form of the English word 'spirit' is the term 'spiritual'. Spirit is a derivative of the Latin word *spiritus*, which also means breath. It has a variety of connotations, and most contrast the material body with an immaterial entity. In metaphysics, the term 'spirit' is frequently used to describe consciousness or personality. In this sense, spirituality and immateriality are synonyms, which may reflect experience of the immanent or transcendent nature of the world, or a belief in immaterial realities. Being spiritual means acting, thinking and engaging from the perspective of being a spirit (immaterial), not a form; as a

N. Pant, *Spirituality, Mental Health and Quality of Life*,
https://doi.org/10.1007/978-981-99-2703-6_1

soul, not a physical body. We develop an awareness of our physical appearance, and we apply labels to our bodies, such as nationality, race, gender and occupation. We are taught to believe that we are our physical forms. Through millennia, the definition of spirituality has evolved. There are differences in how the terms 'spirituality' and 'religion' are used, even though they both refer to the quest for an Absolute or God. Spirituality is sometimes unrelated to any specific religious tradition, but religion indicates a distinct belief and way of life that includes acceptance of a metaphysical or supernatural truth (Lama, 1999). Because the concept of spirituality is widely seen as a type of intelligence in psychology, this chapter also presents a brief summary of spiritual intelligence (SQ).

1.2 Spiritual Intelligence (SQ)

In earlier investigations, the two terms 'spirituality' and 'religiosity' have sometimes been taken as the same idea. The utilization of the term 'spirituality' has changed from time to time. The comparability between the terms 'spirituality' and 'religiosity' is that both identify an outright or higher cognizance, yet even there we discover contrasts in their utilization. Religiosity infers a specific custom of belief that incorporates acknowledgement of spiritual or heavenly reality (Lama, 1999), while spirituality isn't bound to a specific religious convention. Religiosity is related to formal association, yet spirituality does not rely upon any institutional alliance. Religiosity demonstrates an organized approach to identifying with circumstances, occasions and individuals. Spirituality works in a more individualized way. It is inherent and picked by an individual, while religiosity may be viewed as the main thrust. Religiosity is likely to be identified with Christianity, Islam, Hinduism, Buddhism and so forth. Spirituality is an individual method for identifying with the Divine, the self, individuals, and the world. Today, in psychology the idea of spirituality is becoming the focus of study as a type of intelligence. Once, the idea of intelligence was viewed completely in the light of legitimate and numerical capacities. Thus, initially, it was assumed that IQ would be a reliable predictor of professional success. In fact, it has turned out to be a relatively poor gauge of potential advancement. Now, it appears that IQ is the criteria that requires the fewest requirements to be considered for a top position. What motivates success when one has chosen a vocation definitely remains murky. Pondering this has fuelled psychologists' interest in emotional intelligence (EQ), a concept made prominent by Daniel Goleman in his book in the middle of the 1990s. Moreover, the investigation continues because a computer may have a greater IQ than humans, and other creatures can also have EQ (i.e., the capacity to comprehend one's own feelings and the feelings of others). It is possessing the capacity of spiritual intelligence (SQ) to address the issue of life's purpose and values that distinguishes humans from other living things on the planet (Zohar & Marshall, 2000). Spiritual intelligence encourages us to ask big questions like, Why was I born? What purpose does my life serve? Why am I dedicating my life to this partnership, this endeavour, or this cause? What exactly am I trying to achieve in this task or in my life? It allows us to get a fuller picture and to see the larger context in which things take place. It infuses our lives with a profound sense of meaning and value (Zohar & Marshall, 2004). Simply put, spiritual intelligence is the manifestation of our intrinsic spiritual traits in our ideas, deeds and attitudes. In psychology, SQ describes the ultimate level of intellect, which comes after IQ and EQ. According to Danah Zohar, SQ is what we employ to cultivate our capacity for, and desire for, meaning, vision and value. Spiritual intelligence encourages communication between the mind and the body as well as between reason and emotion. It enables us to bridge the distance between the self and other and integrate the intrapersonal and interpersonal. Spiritual intelligence, according to Vaughan (2002), is concerned with the interior life of the mind and spirit and how it relates to being in the world. Furthermore, according to Amram and Dryer (2008), spiritual intelligence is the capacity to utilize, embody and manifest spiritual resources, values and attributes to improve daily functioning and wellbeing.

1.3 Religiosity

Religiosity is a set of beliefs and faith about the ultimate truth. In Indian psychology, religiosity holds a slightly different meaning based only on belief or faith. Religiosity ('dharma') in Indian psychology (philosophy) is the science of acquiring the ultimate truth. Religiosity is the source or way ('sadhan') to acquire the ultimate truth or goal ('sadhya'), or reality or spirituality ('adhyatmikta'). The state of being religious is what the term 'religiosity' refers to. The adjectival form the word 'religion' is 'religious'. *Oxford Dictionaries* (n.d.-a) defines the term religious as being connected to or believing in a particular religion. Regarding 'religion', this is a derivation of the Latin verb *religo/religare*, meaning to bind, as in to bind ourselves to the worship of the one true God. Thus, the term 'religion' refers to the adoration of a personal deity or gods and the belief in their supreme authority (Oxford Dictionaries, n.d.-b). In order to put it another way, religion can be defined as an organized set of beliefs, cultural norms and worldviews that connect people to the divine and spirituality.

1.4 Mental Health

Because of social factors and different ideas on mental health, a consistent definition is difficult to locate. Psychological well-being or the absence of a mental disorder are possible ways to define mental health. According to positive psychology a person's capacity to enjoy life, and to strike a balance between daily activities and efforts to develop resilience is a measure of the mental health. An effective adaptability to a range of challenges and the expression of emotions are other further descriptions of mental health. According to the World Health Organization (WHO), mental health is a state of wellbeing marked by self-awareness, the ability to manage everyday stresses, the capacity for productive and fruitful work and the capacity to contribute to one's community. *The American Heritage Dictionary of the English Language* (2009) defines mental health as a condition of emotional and psychological wellbeing in which a person can use their cognitive and emotional capacities, participate in society and meet the regular demands of daily living. Or to put it another way, a person's overall emotional and psychological state is referred to as their mental health. As far as the term 'mental illness' is concerned, a disorder that impairs a person's cognitive, social, emotional or behavioural state or abilities is generally considered to be mental illness (American Psychiatric Association, 2000). There are several ways to understand the idea of 'normality' if we look at it carefully:

1. *Health as normality*: According to this definition, which is shared by both conventional medical-psychiatric terminology and common usage, normality is simply the absence of illness.
2. *Normality as ideal*: The goal is to define normality in terms of an ideal or desired state, and includes those that stress the significance of achieving a positive mental state (e.g., Jahoda, 1958) or the goals of psychological growth, such as self-actualization (Goldstein, 1939; Maslow, 1954), in becoming a fully functional person (Rogers, 1963), or forming a mature personality (Allport, 1961).
3. *Normality as average*: The statistics of measurement on the normal probability curve provide a third perspective on normalcy.
4. *Normality as socially acceptable*: The concept of normality here is seen as something that is socially acceptable and maintains that behaviour can only be judged in terms of the social context in which it occurs. If it adheres to societal norms, it is regarded as normal; if not, it is viewed as deviant or abnormal.
5. *Normality as process*: This viewpoint seeks to define normality in terms of processes throughout time, as opposed to addressing it from a cross-sectional perspective.

If we take a look at Indian psychology, we find plenty of information on mental health (Manasik Swasthya). According to the Charaka Samhita (Sutra 1/ 56) '"Vata", "pitta" and "kapha" are physical disorders and "rajoguna" and "tamoguna" are mental disorders.' Similarly, in the Mahabharata mental health is defined as follows:

> सत्वं रजस्तम इति मानसाः स्युस्त्रयो गुणाः
>
> satvam rajastam iti maanasaah syustrayo gunaah,
>
> तेषां गुणानां साम्यं यत्त दाहुः स्वस्थलक्षणम्
>
> tesam gunanam saamyam yakt daahuh swasthlakshanam.
>
> 'Sattva', 'raja' and 'tama' are three mental traits. The balancing state of the three traits is the state of actual mental health.
>
> (Mahabharata, Santiparva 16/13)

1.5 Quality of Life

In discussing quality of life, the WHO is the leading authority to describe and define it. The concept of quality of life (QoL) usually includes subjective evaluations of both positive and negative aspects of life (WHOQOL, 1998). The WHO in the WHOQOL-BREF suggested four domains of QoL. The first is *physical health* which incorporates activities of daily living, dependence on medicinal substances and medical aids, energy/fatigue, mobility, pain/discomfort, sleep/rest, and work capacity. The second domain, *psychological health*, incorporates bodily image and appearance, negative feelings, positive feelings, self-esteem, spirituality/religion/personal beliefs, thinking, learning, memory and concentration. The third, *social relationships*, includes personal relationships, social support and sexual issues. Finally, the fourth domain, *environment*, includes financial resources, freedom, physical safety and security, health and social care (accessibility and quality), home environment, opportunities for acquiring new information and skills, participation in and opportunities for recreation and leisure activities, physical environment (pollution/noise/traffic/climate) and transport. As stated by the WHOQOL Group (1994a, 1994b): 'Quality of life is defined as individuals' perceptions of their position in life within the context of the culture and value systems in which they live and in relation to their goals, expectations, standards, and concerns.'

1.6 Spirituality/Religiosity and Mental Health

Some research studies indicate the relationship between the dimensions of spirituality and mental health, as follows. By conducting a meta-analysis, Bergin (1983) discovered that religion is a multidimensional phenomenon with both positive and negative characteristics. According to Adams et al. (2000), the influence of life purpose on perceived wellness is mediated by optimism and a sense of coherence, and it also has independent effects on perceived wellness that go beyond the influence of life purpose. Faith was shown to have the strongest link with good mental health, according to Meisenhelder and Chandler (2002). In a subsequent study on US college students, Nagel and Sgoutas-Emch (2007) discovered that those with higher spirituality scores were more active and had different health views than those with lower spirituality scores. According to research by Allen et al. (2008), having more everyday spiritual encounters and not feeling abandoned by God were linked to greater emotional health. A substantial correlation between spiritual intelligence and happiness was discovered by Faribors et al. (2010) among Iranian nurses. Spirituality has been identified by Koenig (2010) as a psychological and social resource for dealing with stress. According to Abadi et al. (2012), spiritual intelligence was higher in a fasting group than it was in non-fasting groups, either without an excuse or with an excuse. It was also higher in the non-fasting groups with an excuse than it was in the non-fasting groups without an excuse. Isfahani and Nobakht (2013) discovered a strong positive link between employee happiness and spiritual intelligence. According to Shojaei and Ghaffari (2013), there is a considerable correlation between religious practices, religious decisions and religious life choices, as well as spiritual intelligence and its components (transcendental consciousness, spiritual experiences, forgiveness). According to Alihosseini et al. (2014), inner peace, spiritual experiences, forgiveness, and self-recognition, all components of spiritual intelligence, have a positive and significant link with happiness. According to Singh et al. (2010), the significant predictors of mental health are the type of school, spiritual intelligence, altruism, rejection (a component of the school environment) and control (a dimension of the school environment).

1.7 Spirituality/Religiosity and Quality of Life

The following research studies indicate the relationship between spirituality and its dimensions and QoL. Fehring et al. (1987) found a weak positive relationship between life changes and depression. Koenig (2004) found spirituality related to better mental health, greater wellbeing, and greater QoL. In their study, Teichmann et al. (2006) discovered a strong correlation between the WHOQOL-100 spirituality score and the quality-of-life index. Additionally, it was discovered that spirituality was linked to all aspects of quality of life (physical health, psychological wellbeing, level of independence, social relationships and environment). According to Hsu et al. (2009) religion and spirituality has a substantial positive correlation with international students' psychological and social quality of life. Bolghan-Abadi et al. (2014) found spiritual intelligence played an effective role in predicting quality of life. Khan et al. (2011), in their study carried out in India, found spirituality to be a positive significant predictor of life satisfaction, and a positive correlation between spirituality and life satisfaction. Singh and Sinha (2013) found greater QoL in most cases where SQ was high. Kaur and Kaur (2014) found high levels of organizational spirituality in employees leading to job satisfaction, a higher quality of work life and lower occupational stress.

1.8 The Role of Spirituality/Religiosity in Alleviating Mental Illness and Enhancing Quality of Life

As observed earlier, there is considerable evidence showing positive relationships between spirituality/religiosity and mental/overall health. In a recent study by Pant and Srivastava (2019), it was discovered that a significant relationship between spiritual intelligence and mental health exists among both arts and science students, and that there is a significant correlation between spiritual intelligence and mental health for both male and female arts and science students separately. Additionally, Pant and

Srivastava (2015) reported a significant relationship between spiritual intelligence and quality of life in both male and female arts and science students, as well as a significant relationship between spiritual intelligence and quality of life in both groups of students (combined). Pant and Srivastava (2014), in further research, found that spiritual intelligence and mental health had a significant correlation, that there was a significant relationship between spiritual intelligence and quality of life, and finally, that there was a significant relationship between mental health and quality of life among college students involved in the study. In a review of research, by Elmer et al. (2003), it was found that spiritually oriented people seem to respond better to intervention and handle trauma better when facing an injury, (Emmons, 2000), and spiritually oriented people have lower depression rates (MacDonald & Friedman, 2002). Further, Trott (1996) indicated a positive correlation between spiritual wellbeing and general self-efficacy.

On the basis of this analysis and review it can be summarized that spirituality and related constructs are one of the most powerful predictors of mental health and quality of life. Also, spirituality and related constructs have a positive relationship with mental health and quality of life. There is a need for more scientific and stable conceptions in the field of mental health to support effective treatment. To this end, effort has been made both in this chapter and the rest of the book, in searching the pathways of Indian psychology.

1.9 Health, Mental Health and Mind in Indian Psychology

Indian psychology defines health ('swasthya') as an Ayurvedic approach indicating health as a balance in the three 'doshas' (Vata, pitta, and kapha the three bodily humors), thirteen 'agni' (flames or metabolic fires), seven 'dhatus' (tissues), and in the processes of eliminating waste products. Finally, health is defined as the contentment of the 'atma' (soul or consciousness), the five senses and the mind:

> समदोषः समाग्निश्च समधातुमलक्रियः।
>
> Samdosah samagnisch samdhatumalkriyah,
>
> प्रसन्नात्मेन्द्रियमनाः स्वस्थ इत्यभिधीयते।।
>
> Prasannatmendriyamana swasth ityabhidheeyate.
>
> Balance in 'vata', 'pitta' and 'kapha' ('doshas'), flames or metabolic fires ('agni'), tissues ('dhatu'), processes of eliminating waste products ('malkriya') and happiness of soul or consciousness ('atma') and senses is called health ('swasthya').
>
> [Shushruta Samhita, 15/41]

According to Ayurveda, good health is a balance of both biological and psychological factors. The Raamcharitmana*s*, a well-known text, describes three major mental illnesses: 'kama' (false desire), 'krodha' (anger), and 'lobha' (greed), which are brought on by an imbalance of the three 'tridoshas': 'vata', 'pitta' and 'kapha'. This definition of health encompasses all facets in this manner. Additionally, three 'gunas' (human natures): 'attva' (the element of illumination), 'rajas' (activity and dynamism), and 'amas' (passivity, darkness), need to be in balance in order for a person to be in good health. The Bhagvad Gita frequently states that this balanced condition of functioning is what constitutes a person's psychological well-being (Palsane et al., 1986; Sinha, 1990). According to Ayurveda, mental health is a condition of mental, intellectual and spiritual well-being. The three previously mentioned mental illnesses are caused by 'rajas guna', according to the Bhagvad Gita (Gita, 3/37). In addition to this, we have a wealth of information on spirituality and mental/physical health from an Indian perspective in the form of the Charaka Samhita, Sushruta Samhita, further Ayurvedic works, Sad-Darshana, and numerous other volumes. 'Vata', 'pitta' and 'kapha' are three bodily ailments, and 'rajas' and 'tamas' are two mental disorders, according to Charaka Samhita (Sutra Sthan). The third 'sattva guna', according to Charaka Rishi, is a good nature required for mental health rather than a problem.

In Indian psychology and Indian philosophy there is a vast quantity of information on health, mental health and related aspects such as Yoga, Upanishads, Gita and Vedanta among others. *Patanjali Yoga Sutra* is a leading book by Mahamuni Patanjali, which describes the psychological concepts along with their clinical use. The famous 'root sutra' of *Patanjali Yoga Sutra* is where yoga is explained as:

> योगश्च चित्तवृत्ति निरोध:
>
> Yogashchittavrittinirodhah.
>
> Yoga is restraining the mind-stuff ('chitta') from taking various forms ('vrttis').
>
> [1 – Patanjali Yoga Sutra, 1/2]

When discussing the character of Shree Krishna, we see it is full of psychological phenomena. When Arjuna denied fighting the war against his relatives in Kurukshetra then Bhagwan Shree Krishna blessed him with the 'Gita Gyan' to fight with his negative mindset up. That is why Gita is also thought of as a therapy (CBT) among Indian psychologists (Sharma, 2014).

A famous saying is: 'No health without mental health' but I would add further: 'No mental health without spiritual health'. Spiritual health comes in life when an individual lives life in spiritual ways. The core and primary school of Indian philosophy is Advaita Vedanta. The Advaita theory is based on the spiritual dimension of wholeness and oneness. And the literature of Swami Shivananda is also full of psychological concepts of mind and Indian psychology. He has represented Indian psychology worldwide. Swami Shivananda (2005) in his book *Manojay* explained that there are three types of the feeling of self:

> Saatvika Ahankara: To feel as I am Brahma.
>
> Rajsika Ahankara: To feel like I am a king, or intelligent.
>
> Taamsika Ahankara: To feel I am fool, or know nothing.

According to Indian philosophy, the root cause of all troubles is 'ahankaara' (feeling of self). And the aim of all Gyan, Karma, and Bhakti Yoga is to be free from this 'ahankara' or feeling of self. Swami Shivananda Ji further explained 'ahankara' as twofold:

Sthool Ahankara: To feel oneself as a body.

Sooksma Ahankara: To have this feeling of 'ahankara' about any theory or school.

On the basis of all the discussion, it may be concluded that the concept of mental health is as perfectly and effectively defined in Indian psychology as in other approaches and may be used in future scholastic and applied purposes. For this we need more scientific and stronger approaches on all these mentioned constructs, which are explored in the following chapters.

References

Abadi, M. Z. B., Farid, A. A. A., Bahari, F., & Chami, M. (2012). The effect of Islamic fasting in Quran on spiritual intelligence and happiness of fasting persons. *Quran Medicine, 1*(3), 66–70.

Adams, T. B., Bezner, J. R., Drabbs, M. E., Zambarano, R. J., & Steinhardt, M. A. (2000). Conceptualization and measurement of the spiritual and psychological dimensions of wellness in a college population. *Journal of American College Health, 48*(4), 165–173.

Alihosseini, F., Rangan, U., Alihosseini, A., & Hajmohammadi, F. (2014). A study of the relationship between spiritual intelligence and its components with happiness in youths. *The International Journal of Humanities & Social Studies, 2*(6), 56–60.

Allen, R. S., Phillips, L. L., Roff, L. L., Cavanaugh, R., & Day, L. (2008). Religiousness/spirituality and mental health among older male inmates. *The Gerontologist, 48*(5), 692–697.

Allport, G. W. (1961). *Pattern and growth in personality*. Holt, Rinehart and Winston.

American Psychiatric Association. (2000). *Diagnostic and statistical manual of mental disorders* (4th ed.). Author.

Amram, Y., & Dryer, D. C. (2008, August). *The Integrated Spiritual Intelligence Scale (ISIS): Development and preliminary validation*. Paper Presented at the 116th Annual Conference of the American Psychological Association.

Bergin, A. E. (1983). Religiosity and mental health: A critical re-evaluation and meta-analysis. *Professional Psychology: Research and Practice, 14*(2), 170–184.

Bolghan-Abadi, M., Ghofrani, F., & Abde-Khodaei, M. S. (2014). Study of the spiritual intelligence role in predicting university students' quality of life. *Journal of Religion and Health, 53*(1), 79–85.

Elmer, L., MacDonald, D., & Friedman, H. (2003). Transpersonal psychology, physical health, and mental health: Theory, research and practice. *Humanistic Psychologist, 31*, 159–181.

Emmons, R. A. (2000). Is spirituality an intelligence? *The International Journal for the Psychology of Religion, 10*, 27–34.

Faribors, B., Fatemeh, A., & Hamidreza, H. (2010). The relationship between nurses' spiritual intelligence and happiness in Iran. *Procedia Social and Behavioral Sciences, 5*, 1556–1561.

Fehring, R. J., Brennan, P. F., & Keller, M. L. (1987). Psychological and spiritual well-being in college students. *Research in Nursing & Health, 10*(6), 391–398.

Goldstein, K. (1939). *The organism*. American Book Company.

Hsu, P. H., Krägeloh, C. U., Shepherd, D., & Billington, R. (2009). Religion/spirituality and quality of life of international tertiary students in New Zealand: An exploratory study. *Mental Health, Religion & Culture, 12*(4), 385–399.

Isfahani, A. N., & Nobakht, M. (2013). Impact of spiritual intelligence on the staff happiness (Case study: Golpayegan Petrochemical Company). *International Journal of Academic Research in Business and Social Sciences, 3*(7), 253–266.

Jahoda, M. (1958). *Current concepts of positive mental health*. Basic Books.

Kaur, M., & Kaur, D. (2014). The power of organizational spirituality: Its effect on job satisfaction, quality of work life and occupational stress. *International Journal of Research in Organizational Behavior and Human Resource Management, 2*(2), 356–369.

Khan, M. A., Shirazi, M., & Ahmed, M. (2011). Spirituality and life satisfaction among adolescents in India. *Journal of Subcontinent Researches, 3*(7), 71–84.

Koenig, H. G. (2004). Spirituality, wellness, and quality of life. *Sexuality, Reproduction and Menopause, 2*(2), 76–82.

Koenig, H. G. (2010). Spirituality and mental health. *International Journal of Applied Psychoanalytic Studies, 7*(2), 116–122.

Lama, D. (1999). *Ethics for the New Millennium*. Riverhead Books.

MacDonald, D., & Friedman, H. (2002). Assessment of humanistic, transpersonal and spiritual constructs: State of the science. *Journal of Humanistic Psychology, 42*(4), 102–125.

Maslow, A. H. (1954). *Motivation and personality*. Harper.

Meisenhelder, J. B., & Chandler, E. N. (2002). Spirituality and health outcomes in the elderly. *Journal of Religion and Health, 41*(3), 243–252.

Nagel, E., & Sgoutas-Emch, S. (2007). The relationship between spirituality, health beliefs, and health behaviors in college students. *Journal of Religion and Health, 46*(1), 141–154.

Oxford Dictionaries. (n.d.-a). Retrieved March 2, 2020, from http://oxforddictionaries.com/definition/english/religious?q=religious

Oxford Dictionaries. (n.d.-b). Retrieved March 2, 2020, from http://oxforddictionaries.com/definition/english/religion

Palsane, M. N., Bhavsar, S. N., Goswami, R. P., & Evans, G. W. (1986). The concept of stress in the Indian indicators. *Journal of Indian Psychology, 5*, 1–12.

Pant, N., & Srivastava, S. K. (2014). Effect of spiritual intelligence on mental health and quality of life among college students. *ZENITH International Journal of Multidisciplinary Research, 4*(8), 208–215.

Pant, N., & Srivastava, S. K. (2015). Spiritual intelligence, gender and educational background as related to the quality of life of college students. *Indian Journal of Positive Psychology, 6*(3), 226–232.

Pant, N., & Srivastava, S. K. (2019). The impact of spiritual intelligence, gender and educational background on mental health among college students. *Journal of Religion and Health, 58*, 87–108.

Rogers, C. (1963). The concept of the fully functioning person. *Psychotherapy: Theory, Research and Practice, 1*, 17–26.

Sharma, N. (2014). Cognitive behaviour therapy in perspective of the *Bhagwat Gita*. *International Journal of Humanities and Social Science Invention, 3*(1), 2319–7722.

Shivanand, S. (2005). *Manojay*. Divya Jeevan Sangh.

Shojaei, K., & Ghaffari, S. (2013). The study of the relationship between workers' religious beliefs and spiritual intelligence and general health (Case study: Department of Education of Sardasht). *International Journal of Basic Sciences & Applied Research, 2*(11), 960–967.

Singh, A., Kaur, P., & Singh, T. (2010). Spiritual intelligence, altruism, school environment and academic achievement as predictor of mental health of adolescents. *Journal of Exercise Science and Physiotherapy, 6*(1), 34–38.

Singh, M. P., & Sinha, J. (2013). Impact of spiritual intelligence on quality of life. *International Journal of Scientific and Research Publications, 3*(5), 1–5.

Sinha, D. (1990). Concept of psycho-social well-being: Western and Indian perspectives. *NIMHANS Journal, 8*, 1–11.

Teichmann, M., Murdvee, M., & Saks, K. (2006). Spiritual needs and quality of life in Estonia. *Social Indicators Research, 76*(1), 147–163.

The American Heritage Dictionary of the English Language. (2009). Houghton Mifflin Company (4th ed.). http://www.thefreedictionary.com/Mental+health

Trott, D. (1996). *Spiritual wellbeing of workers: An exploratory study of spirituality in the workplace* (Dissertation Abstracts International). University of Texas.

Vaughan, F. (2002). What is spiritual intelligence? *Journal of Humanistic Psychology, 42*(2), 16–33.
WHOQOL. (1998). The world health organization quality of life assessment (WHOQOL): Development and psychometric properties. *Social Science & Medicine, 46*, 1569–1585.
WHOQOL Group. (1994a). Development of the WHOQOL: Rationale and current status. *International Journal of Mental Health, 23*(3), 24–56.
WHOQOL Group. (1994b). The development of the World Health Organization quality of life assessment instrument (the WHOQOL). In J. Orley & W. Kuyken (Eds.), *Quality of life assessment: international perspectives.* Springer Verlag.
Zohar, D., & Marshall, I. (2000). *Spiritual intelligence: The ultimate intelligence.* Bloomsbury.
Zohar, D., & Marshall, I. (2004). *Spiritual capital: Wealth we can live by.* Berrett-Koehler Publishers.

Chapter 2
Spirituality, Mental Health and Quality of Life: An Introduction

No health without mental health and no mental health without spiritual health.

Author

2.1 Spirituality

The term 'spirituality' seems at first to be like religiosity. In general parlance, a person who engages with regular religious practices may be called religious or spiritual. But there is some difference between the terms 'spiritual' and 'religious'. What is obvious and undisputed within the meaning of spirituality, is that it comes from the base word 'spirit'. The suffix '-uality' qualifies the utilization of spirit. The *Free Dictionary* (n.d.-a) defines spirituality as the state, quality, manner or fact of being spiritual. Its root word 'spirit' derives from the Latin *spiritus*, meaning 'breath'. It has other common connotations such as spirit, soul, courage and vigour, which come from a Proto-Indo-European word (Calvert, 2000). If one examines the various meanings of the word 'spirit,' they are often found to be contrasted with the material body, or in other words, to mean something immaterial. The non-physical portion of a person that holds emotions and character, sometimes known as the soul, is referred to as the person's 'spirit', according to *Oxford Dictionaries* (n.d.-a). This allows us to define spirit as an immaterial concept. From different viewpoints, the term 'spirituality' may be used in a variety of ways. In an Internet search for the meaning of spirituality today, we discover a large number of entries. According to *Dictionary.com* (n.d.), spirituality is: (1) the quality or fact of being spiritual; (2) incorporeal or immaterial nature; (3) predominantly spiritual character as shown in thought, life, spiritual tendency or tone; or (4) often, spiritualities, property, or revenue of the church or an ecclesiastic in his or her official capability. From *Living Words of Wisdom* (n.d.) we discover: 'The definition of spirituality is that which relates to or affects the human spirit or soul as opposed to material or physical things'. From the *Order of Time.com* (n.d.), we find this entry: 'spirituality is something deeply religious, something relating to the spirit and sacred matters.' What is the fundamental definition of spirituality,

N. Pant, *Spirituality, Mental Health and Quality of Life*,
https://doi.org/10.1007/978-981-99-2703-6_2

then? The quality of one's sensitivity to spiritual things might be used as a basic definition of spirituality. And what are these spiritual things? These are things like love, justice, peace and other things that cannot be immediately sensed by our senses but whose effects can be inferred or calculated from our observations. The assumption that we prefer to view people and/or the rest of creation as consisting of something immaterial, invisible and beyond the realm of current knowledge is fundamental to the way that spirituality is now understood. What we can understand with our senses and with our reason is always expanding. The term 'spirituality' refers to all that cannot be directly perceived with the eyes, directly understood by the senses, or that can only be recognized by reason. In this sense, spirituality and immateriality are synonyms. This is spirituality in the truest sense of the word.

After Danah Zohar's (2000) works on spiritual intelligence, it is now clear that the ideas of spirituality and religiosity are not the same as they were in earlier studies in the field of psychology. Spirituality is now taken to be a trait of searching for the meaning and purpose in life. Some of the more prevalent themes in the literature describe it by utilizing one or more of the following areas: a sense of purpose; a sense of connectedness to self, others, nature, God, or the Other (Hassed, 2000); a quest for wholeness (Humphreys, 2000); a search for hope or harmony (McSherry, 2000); or a belief in a higher being or beings (Hassed, 2000), Some level of transcendence, or the awareness that life consists of more than just the material or practical (Oldnall, 1996) and the pursuits that give people's lives meaning and value. According to Tisdell (2003), spirituality is a crucial aspect of the human experience and is essential to understanding how people come to form meaningful knowledge. According to Tisdell, spirituality has a significant cultural component that influences intellectual growth. The cultural context is where meaning-making takes place and where it is mediated. Spirituality is the idea of an ultimate or purportedly immaterial reality, a personal journey leading to self-discovery, or the deepest values and meanings by which people live (Sheldrake, 2007). Many people see spirituality as a source of inspiration or direction in life (Waaijman, 2002). It can encompass belief in immaterial realities or experiences of the immanent or transcendent nature of the world. As previously mentioned, the terms 'spirituality' and 'religiosity' have diversified in their uses over time. While the terms 'spirituality' and 'religion' each relate to the exploration of an Absolute or God, there are variations in their usage. According to Lama (1999), religion implies a specific faith tradition that accepts the existence of a metaphysical or supernatural reality. In contrast, spirituality need not be connected to any particular religious tradition.

Spirituality from an Indian perspective: The English word 'spirituality' translates as 'aadhyatmikta' (आध्यात्मिकता) in Hindi. The word 'aadhyatm' is made of two words 'adhi' + 'atma', where 'adhi' means owner/controller ('adhisthata') and 'atma' is used here in the sense of one's own body. In this way, the meaning of 'aadhyatmik' refers to that knowledge that is related to the controller/owner/beholder of the body.

In Indian philosophy, we find clear evidence of the word 'aadhyatmikta' as 'aadhyatmopnishad', a part of Shukla Yajurveda. 'Aadhyatmopnishad' broadly explores the concept of ‘aatm tatva’ (self). Apart from this, all Upnishads explore spiritual (‘aadhyatmik’) knowledge.

2.1.1 *Religiosity*

The quality of being religious is indicated by the word ‘religiosity’. The adjectival form of the word ‘religion’ is ‘religious’. The definition of ‘religious’ in the *Oxford Dictionaries* (n.d.-b) is related to or believing in a religion. Generally, religiosity is based on faith tradition. Furthermore, the word ‘religion’ is a derivation of the Latin verb *religo (religare)*, which means to tie, as in to bind oneself to the worship of the one true God. That is why religion refers to the adoration of a personal god or gods and the belief in a superhuman ruling force (Oxford Dictionaries, n.d.-c). To put it another way, religion can be defined as an organized set of beliefs, cultural norms and worldviews that connect to the supernatural and spirituality. Definitions of religion can also have some restrictions that are either too strict or unclear. We require a definition that encompasses the substance of what religion means across cultural boundaries, taking into account social, psychological and historical variables, and allowing for more expansive grey regions when considering religion in order to avoid these constraints.

Religiosity from an Indian perspective: The word ‘religion’ is different from the Hindi word ‘dharma’ (धर्म). Where religion means binding in the faith, on the other hand, ‘dharma’ means ‘holding virtues’ which leads to the ultimate truth or god. The word ‘dharma’ is made of the root word ‘dhri’ (धृ धारणे) by affixing ‘man’ (मन्). Based on these words’ meanings, ‘dharma’ is ‘which holds’ or which is ‘to be held.’ So, furthermore, it could be stated that the qualities which virtuous people hold are called ‘dharma’. The *Manu Smriti*, a famous theological text of India, identifies ten characteristics of ‘dharma’:

> धृति: क्षमा दमोऽस्तेयं शौचमिन्द्रियनिग्रह: ।
> Dhriti chhayama damosteyam sauchmindriyanigrah
>
> धीर्विद्या सत्यमक्रोधो दशकं धर्मलक्षणम् ।।
> Dheervidyaa satyamkrodho dashkam dharmalakchhanam.
>
> (1) ‘dhriti’ (patience), (2) ‘kshama’ (forgiveness, and also doing favours to one’s abuser), (3) ‘dum’ (always indulging in righteousness with restraint), (4) ‘astheya’ (not stealing), (5) ‘sauch’ (defecation, inner and outer purity), (6) ‘indriya nigrah’ (keeping control over senses, indulging senses always in ‘dharmacharan’), (7) ‘dhee’ (increasing the intellect by virtue), (8) ‘vidya’ (gaining real knowledge), (9) ‘satyam’ (always conducting truth), and (10)’akrodha’ (giving up anger and always being calm).
>
> Manu Smriti, 6/91

2.1.2 *Differences Between Spirituality and Religiosity*

As mentioned earlier, both of the terms 'spirituality' and 'religiosity' have been used interchangeably in past studies and research. The definition of spirituality has frequently changed. Although there are distinctions in their applications, there is a connection between the terms 'spirituality' and 'religiosity' in that both pertain to the search for an absolute or higher consciousness. According to Lama (1999), religion denotes a certain faith tradition that accepts the existence of a metaphysical or supernatural reality, whereas spirituality is not necessarily associated with any one particular faith. Where spirituality is personal, intrinsic, and chosen by an individual, religiosity, on the other hand, is concerned with a traditional affiliation such as Christianity, Islam, Hinduism and Buddhism, among others. Today, in psychological research the concept of spirituality is studied as a form of intelligence: spiritual intelligence (SQ). According to Danah Zohar and Ian Marshall (2000), developers of the concept of spiritual intelligence (SQ):

> Traditional religion is a set of beliefs imposed from others. It is top-down, passed down through the family and tradition or absorbed from monks, prophets, and holy texts. A raw ability of the human brain and mind, SQ (spiritual intelligence) draws its most profound resources from the centre of the universe itself. It is a capability that the brain has developed over countless years that allows it to look for and apply meaning while solving challenges.

As far as Indian psychology is concerned, it too, expresses religiosity as a set of virtues and devotion to spiritual and physical wellbeing, but considers spirituality as related to ultimate and eternal truth and cause of being. Religiosity is a way to get spirituality. Therefore, religiosity is the form of means and spirituality is the goal. Table 2.1 indicates the key differences between spirituality and religiosity.

2.2 Spiritual Intelligence

Once it was commonly held that students with good study skills would take the science stream, those with fewer study skills would take the commerce stream, and those with even fewer skills would take the arts stream, while those with the fewest skills would take nothing and become hermits or religious leaders. More recently, this has become a joke because highly skilled students taking the science stream (e.g., engineers) may work under the commerce stream (e.g., HR, MBA); commerce stream students may later work under arts stream students (e.g., administrators); and administrators may work under politicians with very few study skills. And finally, all these people with study skills, especially politicians, work as per the very least skilled people such as Sants, Father, Maulavi, and other religious heads. Why do such things happen? This leads our attention to the concepts of PQ, IQ, EQ, and SQ. A person with PQ (physical intelligence) could become a good athlete or sports person, but animals could also have good PQ. A person with IQ (cognitive intelligence) could

Table 2.1 Comparing religiosity and spirituality

Religiosity	Spirituality
1. Religiosity is associated with formal organization	1. Spirituality does not depend on institutional affiliation
2. Religiosity is indicative of a particular faith tradition	2. Spirituality is not bound to any particular religious tradition
3. Religiosity may be related to Christianity, Hinduism, Buddhism, Islam, etc	3. It is a personal method of relating to the divine, oneself, other people, and the world is through spirituality
4. Religiosity denotes a structured approach to interacting with the divine	4. Spirituality operates in a personal way
5. Religiosity sometimes acts as a driving force	5. It is intrinsic and chosen by an individual
6. Religion may be inherited from monks, religious heads, holy books, family and tradition	6. Spirituality is an innate individual ability
7. It is based on faith tradition	7. It is based on a rationale
8. As per Indian psychology, religiosity is the means to get the divinity	8. As per Indian psychology, spirituality is an ultimate goal of these means

be a good engineer or mathematician, but a computer could also have good IQ. A person with EQ (emotional intelligence) could be a good politician or counsellor, but an animal could also have good EQ. The only thing which is unique and specific in human beings is SQ (spiritual intelligence) which only a human being, particularly a spiritual person, can have.

The term IQ was coined by German psychologist William Stern in 1912 and later developed by Alfred Binet. The concept of EQ was primarily defined by Peter Salovey and John Mayer and later popularized by Daniel Goleman with his book, published in 1995, titled Emotional Intelligence. In 1997, Danah Zohar introduced the concept of spiritual intelligence in her book, Rewriting the Corporate Brain.

In my opinion, simply put, intelligence is the ability to solve problems. As has already been mentioned, the original definition of intelligence placed a strong emphasis on logical and mathematical skills. Initially, it was thought that IQ would be a reliable indicator of career success. However, it has proven to be a poor indicator of success. By all accounts, IQ appears to be associated with the fewest requirements for entering a job. Once you have chosen your profession, it is clear that there are many different factors that contribute to your success. This phenomenon has drawn psychologists' focus onto another type of intelligence that people need in life: emotional intelligence (EQ), which Daniel Goleman first introduced in his book of the same name in the middle of the 1990s. Despite this, research continues since computers may be smarter than people and animals may also possess emotional intelligence (EQ) (the ability to understand one's own and others' emotions). Something special exists in the world that distinguishes humans from other organisms; this is their spiritual intelligence (SQ), their capacity to grapple with the issues of life's value and meaning (Zohar & Marshall, 2000). The most basic queries raised by SQ are: Why was I born? What purpose does my life serve? Why am I dedicating my life to this friendship, career or cause? Spiritual intelligence enables us to get a broader perspective on events and their wider context. It provides a vast canopy of meaning and value for our lives (Zohar & Marshall, 2004). SQ is exclusively human and the most fundamental of the three; unlike IQ, which computers possess, and EQ, which occurs in higher animals (Zohar & Marshall, 2000), SQ enables us to have vision and meaning. It enables us to aspire and dream. It serves as the foundation for the beliefs we tend to hold as well as the influence our values and beliefs have on the activities we perform. It is the essence of being human and is viewed as an ultimate intelligence. We have a desire to place our lives in some larger, meaning-giving context, be it family, the community, work, a religious framework or the universe itself. This takes us far beyond the current moment and ourselves. Spiritual intelligence permits individuals to be artistic, to vary the rules and to change the scenario by extending the boundaries. It makes us the full intellectual, emotional and spiritual creatures that we are. So, it has no necessary connection with religion. Finally, SQ is the ultimate intelligence living on the top end of the hierarchy of PQ, IQ, and EQ. After the emergence of the third force in psychology as a humanistic approach, this is the next step to this approach in positive and transpersonal psychology.

The following are examples of indications of a highly developed spiritual intelligence (SQ), according to Zohar and Marshall's (2000) book *Spiritual Intelligence: The Ultimate Intelligence*:

- The capacity to be flexible or actively and spontaneously adaptive
- Possessing a great level of self-awareness and the ability to accept and bear pain
- The ability to confront and overcome pain
- The capacity to be motivated by purpose and values
- The ability to motivate people
- A desire to avoid harm that is not necessary
- A propensity for seeing the relationships among various things or being 'holistic'
- A noticeable propensity to question why
- Having the capacity to go against the grain.

Spiritual intelligence, according to Emmons (1999), is 'a framework for identifying and classifying the skills and abilities required for the adaptive application of spirituality'. Emmons (2000) suggests these four characteristics of spiritual intelligence: (1) the capacity to draw on spiritual resources to address problems; (2) the capacity to access states of heightened consciousness; (3) the capacity to view commonplace interactions and activities with a sense of the sacred; and (4) the capacity to transcend the physical and material. According to Vaughan (2002), spiritual intelligence is 'the capacity for a deep understanding of existential issues and insight into several levels of consciousness. It suggests knowledge of our interconnectedness with the transcendent, one another, the earth, and all living things'. Zohar and Marshall (2000) define spiritual intelligence as:

> the intelligence with which we address and solve issues of meaning and value, the intelligence with which we are able to place our actions and our lives in a wider, richer, meaning-giving context, the intelligence with which we can assess that one course of action or one life-path is more meaningful than another.

This definition places an emphasis on the importance of meaning. According to Levin (2000), we demonstrate spiritual intelligence when we live in a way that incorporates spirituality into our everyday life. According to Wolman (2001), spiritual intelligence is 'the human ability to raise ultimate issues regarding the meaning of existence and to simultaneously experience the seamless affiliation between each of us and the world in which we live'. According to Nasel (2004), having spiritual intelligence refers to

> the capacity to more effectively recognize, find meaning in, and address existential, spiritual, and practical problems. A person's capacity to find meaning in their experiences, to solve problems, and to improve their capacity for adaptive decision-making should all be facilitated by such resources and abilities, whether they be prayer, intuition, or transcendence.

Cindy Wigglesworth (2006) defines spiritual intelligence as 'the ability to behave with Compassion and Wisdom while maintaining inner and outer peace (equanimity) regardless of the circumstances'. Compassion and wisdom together form the manifestation of love. Her use of 'behave' is vital because it focuses on how well we maintain our centre, stay calm and truly treat others with compassion and knowledge. Her statement of 'regardless of the circumstances' shows that we can maintain our peaceful centre and loving behaviours even under great stress. This is what we tend to admire in our spiritual leaders.

In simple terms, spiritual intelligence is the way that our thoughts, actions and attitudes show our innate spiritual traits. It might be helpful to think about spiritual intelligence as operating on three levels to make it easier to comprehend cognitive, affective and behavioural processes (Dhar et al., 2008).

1. *Cognitive*: It entails looking for answers to existential concerns, exploring the meaning and purpose of life, and working outside of one's own self. It also involves thinking beyond the given circumstances, events and people, as well as considering unrealized possibilities.
2. *Affective*: It examines subjects like empathy, fearlessness, love of nature, healing from jealously, ego anger and death anxiety, as well as participating in music, lyrics, laughing, art, painting, sculpting and dance. It also examines issues like peace and cheerfulness.
3. *Behavioural*: This involves seeking out and engaging in yoga and meditation; cultivating forgiveness, truthfulness and altruism; viewing suffering as a chance for growth; adopting an optimistic view; limiting obsessive material needs; breaking free from inflexible systems; and engaging in preventative health practices.

Zohar and Marshall (2000) discuss a study conducted at the University of California in the 1990s by neurophysiologist Michael Persinger and neurologist V. S. Ramachandran that provided scientific support for SQ. A 'god-spot' has been found to exist in the human brain as a result of this research; it is situated among neuronal connections in the temporal lobes of the brain. During scans with positron emission tomography, these neural areas illuminate whenever the subjects are exposed to discussion of spiritual topics. Of course, this is culture-specific, with Westerners responding to concepts of 'God' and Buddhists and Hindus responding to certain symbols. While the god-spot doesn't prove the existence of God, it will indicate that the brain is programmed to raise elementary queries. This indicates research that tells how the body is connected to spirituality and religiosity. And further, Zohar and Marshall (2004) cited Singer's research on 40 Hz oscillations, which reveals that 40 Hz oscillations are the neural basis for consciousness in the brain. There are many other recent research studies to prove the biological bases of SQ, too.

So, in summary, spiritual intelligence is the ability or capability to solve problems and gain wellbeing with the help of spiritual resources. Spiritual intelligence helps in solving problems whether at cognitive, affective or behavioural levels, or whether concerning the achievement of the highest purposes of life.

2.2.1 *Model or Levels of Four Intelligences (How PQ, IQ, EQ, and SQ Are Related)*

Four distinct cognitive processes; our physical intelligence (PQ), our basic cognitive intelligence (IQ), our emotional intelligence (EQ), and our spiritual intelligence (SQ) are highlighted by the model. For now, we define intelligence (IQ) as the ability to understand the 'what', EQ as the ability to understand the 'how', and SQ as the ability to understand the 'why' of things (Bowell, 2004). The pyramid that follows depicts the development process in the most obvious order (Fig. 2.1).

Wigglesworth (2011) describes this model in her work. As per her model and study, our focus as infants is likely initially to be on body control. Our intelligence quotient (IQ) is currently determined by our linguistic and mental skills, which are also the main topics of our academic studies. We develop certain connection skills early on, but for many of us, EQ, or emotional intelligence, doesn't really take centre stage until after we realize we need to improve, usually in response to criticism in personal and professional interactions. As we begin to seek significance and wonder if this is all there is, SQ, or spiritual intelligence, becomes the centre of attention. There is an association between SQ and EQ. Empathy and some degree of emotional self-awareness are essential building blocks. At that moment, when our spiritual development takes shape, EQ skills begin to be strengthened, which would also strengthen and aid SQ development.

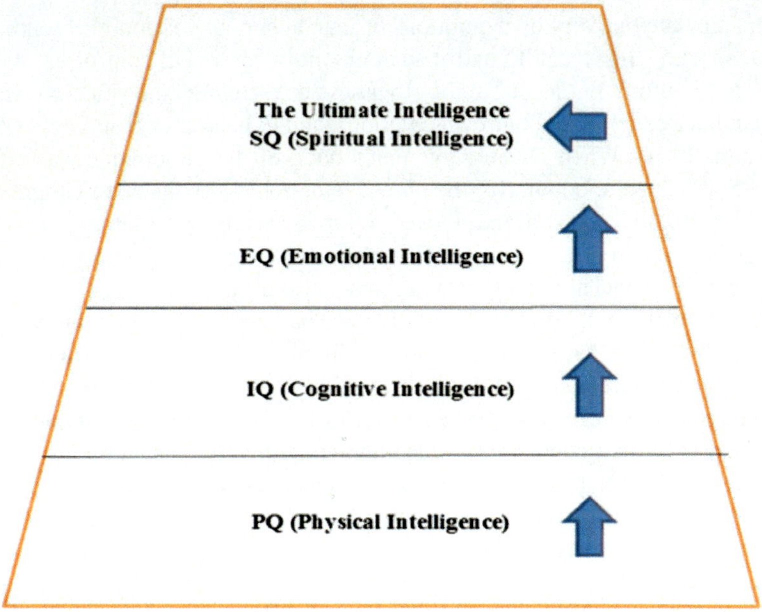

Fig. 2.1 Hierarchy or levels of four intelligences (The image is inspired by Cindy Wigglesworth, 2011)

2.2.2 IQ (What), EQ (How) and SQ (Why)

Intelligence (IQ) 'What': IQ is a type of cognitive intelligence. The French Ministry of Education commissioned Alfred Binet, a psychologist, to construct an official IQ test that would help identify children who were unable to learn as rapidly or as well as others (Ciccarelli & Meyer, 2008). Since 1905, when the first contemporary IQ test was created by Alfred Binet and Theodore Simon, the concept of IQ has become the most discussed and researched matter in studies and research, whether in scholastic or applied fields, and has been seen as a strong predictor of success in life. 'Intelligence quotient' or 'IQ' is generally considered as a measure of analytical or mathematical intelligence. Seven different categories of intelligences were listed by Howard Gardner in his 1983 book *Frames of Mind*, which covered 'multiple intelligences': (1) linguistic; (2) logical-mathematical; (3) musical; (4) bodily-kinesthetic; (5) spatial; (6) interpersonal; and (7) intrapersonal. If we discuss IQ in more scientific way, various research studies also indicate biological evidence. IQ is famously linear. Questions evoke answers in much the same way as neurons seek other neurons. One neuron firing to another to make a neural tract is called synaptic transmission and is the basis for the formal logic of IQ.

Emotional Intelligence (EQ) 'How': Emotional intelligence is intelligence associated with how we relate to and understand other people and the situations within which we stumble upon them. It is also associated with our capability to apprehend and manipulate our very own emotions of fear, anger, aggression or resentment. As Goleman said, 'If we can't control such emotions, they will control us'. Goleman went on to outline EQ as our ability to assess or recognize the situation we are in, to read other people's and our own emotions, and to behave appropriately (Zohar & Marshall, 2004). When Daniel Goleman's book of the same name was published in 1995, it helped to popularize the phrase 'emotional intelligence'. Goleman highlighted Bell Labs' research that looked at top achievers and attempted to ascertain what set them apart from more typical workers. It was thought that top performers had far stronger personal networks and interpersonal skills than typical performance. The work that Goleman wrote about revolutionized our understanding of intelligence and was rapidly seen to have practical application in usual lifestyles and the workplace. Unlike IQ, which remains pretty much constant throughout life, EQ can be nurtured and improved. We can learn to behave extra intelligently in our interactions with other people, or in recognizing and dealing with our very own emotions. Emotional intelligence also somewhat broadened our concept of strategic questioning because it became evident that we pursue emotional strategies as well as rational ones, or, at least, that there is frequently an emotional contribution to the strategies we form. Thus, EQ is different from IQ; it weaves associative patterns. Accessing our EQ is not like gaining access to an answer to a query or doing a mathematical calculation (Bowell, 2004).

Spiritual Intelligence (SQ) 'Why': Science can answer the question of 'what' and can answer the question of 'how', but it cannot answer the question of 'why'. Spirituality can. In essence, everyone has a religious or spiritual orientation. They may pursue different levels of need fulfilment depending on how far they take the growth of such a need. Humanistic psychologist Abraham Maslow grouped these human needs into five categories with a hierarchical structure. In this hierarchy, biological needs like hunger, thirst and sex are at the bottom. Safety requirements that include security, stability and order come next. The next level of belongingness includes identification, affection and attachment. Then comes the need for self-esteem, which includes success, respect for oneself and prestige. The need for self-actualization, which refers to the desire to reach one's full potential in whichever profession one chooses to work in, is the highest level in the hierarchy. Self-actualization is fundamentally spirally cyclic: as a person finds more and more satisfaction, he or she will continue to seek more and more of it. The Indian notion of self-actualization and 'atma sakchaatkaar' are comparable to it. When the term 'ananda' is used in the Vedanta Darshana, it transforms the 'jeeva' (individual self) into the 'parmananda' (universal self). In the materialistic and fiercely competitive world of today, it seems like we are losing both our identity and our sense of purpose. We are under a lot of strain from rapidly advancing technological advancements, and this pressure has made it difficult for us to see other avenues for survival and growth. This leads psychologists' attention to the new, hybridized and burning field of positive and transpersonal psychology, and spiritual intelligence, or SQ—the intellect of the soul. This intelligence is what completes us and makes us whole, and that allows us to integrate the many fragments of our lives, activities and being. 'SQ puts us in touch with the depths of our being and with the deep wells of our potentiality' (Zohar & Marshall, 2004). It makes it possible for knowledge and understanding to rise from the depths of our being to the level of our actions, thoughts, and emotions. SQ also motivates us to advance, and takes us into the unknown and the could-be rather than merely supporting the known or the given. It helps us to behave from higher motives and to have aspirational motivations. When we consider SQ, it is about asking an original question that is unburdened by prior knowledge: Why do we want to be a good father, mother, individual or leader? 'Why' is a procedure of sharing ourselves with the boundless fields of intelligence that we name SQ (Bowell, 2004).

2.2.3 *Comparing IQ, EQ and SQ*

It is necessary to have a look at all three concepts in one place to make comparisons and deepen understanding. Table 2.2 compares and distinguishes the keynotes of all three concepts.

Table 2.2 Comparison of IQ, EQ and SQ

Cognitive intelligence (IQ)	Emotional intelligence (EQ)	Spiritual intelligence (SQ)
1. IQ generally is the ability to solve logical, mathematical and adaptive problems	1. EQ generally is the ability to solve the problems related to one's own and other's emotions	1. SQ generally is the ability to solve the problems of meaning and values
2. The whole or overall ability of a person to act with purpose, think critically, and interact with his surroundings is known as intelligence	2. Emotional intelligence is the capacity or ability to understand one's own emotions, the emotions of others and act appropriately based on these emotions	2. Spiritual intelligence is the capacity to understand the meaning, vision and value of life
3. Calculated by the specific mathematical formula: IQ = MA/CA*100	3. It refers to the non-cognitive and non-physical capacity of the organism. There is currently no specific and well-developed formula to find out the level of EQ	3. It refers to the spiritual and inner self. There is currently no specific formula to quantify SQ
4. About rational, logical and rule-bound thinking	4. About associative, habit bound, pattern-recognizing and emotive thinking	4. About creative, insightful, rule-making, rule-breaking and transformative thinking
5. IQ could get an individual hired	5. EQ could get an individual promoted	5. SQ could get an individual inner peace, tranquillity, real solace and a balanced life
6. Emphasizes learning to know and learning to do	6. Emphasizes learning to live together	6. Emphasizes learning to be
7. IQ relates to and answers the question 'What?'	7. EQ relates to and answers the question 'How?'	7. SQ relates to and answers the question 'Why?'

2.2.4 The Dimensions of Spiritual Intelligence

Amram and Dryer (2008) did a thematic analysis of 71 interviews conducted with participants identified as spiritually intelligent by their colleagues and developed an ecumenical grounded theory of spiritual intelligence. Participants usually identified themselves within major spiritual traditions, which are: Buddhism, Christianity, Hinduism, Islam, Judaism, Non-Dual, Shamanic/Earth, Taoism and Yoga. The ability to employ and incorporate spiritual resources and traits to enhance daily functioning and wellbeing is what they referred to as spiritual intelligence. They discovered seven key characteristics in spiritual intelligence that were almost universal among participants and traditions. These are:

1. *Consciousness*: Mindfulness, spiritual practices, development of refined awareness and self-knowledge, and featuring intuitive trans-rational knowing.
2. *Grace*: The manifestation of gratitude-based trust in, and love for life, as well as living in harmony with the sacred, beauty and joy.
3. *Meaning*: Having a sense of purpose and being called to serve others, even in the face of grief and suffering, giving daily activities importance.
4. *Transcendence*: Compassion, loving-kindness, I-Thou orientation, transcending the distinct egoic self into an interconnected wholeness, as well as the development of interpersonal relationships through empathy.
5. *Truth*: Forgiveness, curiosity, Living in open acceptance and love for all that is (all creation), as well as respect for the wisdom of multiple spiritual traditions.
6. *Peaceful Surrender*: Self-acceptance, inner-wholeness, equanimity, humility, egolessness and peacefully surrendering to a higher-self (God, Truth, Absolute, or true nature).
7. *Inner-directedness*: Discernment, integrity, freedom from conditioning, attachments and fears and inner-freedom aligned in responsible wise action.

Further, Amram (2007) identified 22 capacities under spiritual intelligence and grouped these 22 abilities into five broad domains (which are the first five above-mentioned dimensions) of spiritual intelligence: consciousness, grace, meaning, transcendence and truth. Short descriptions and capabilities under each of the domains are discussed in Chap. 4.

2.2.5 The Operational Definition of Spiritual Intelligence

Spiritual intelligence is used as a construct in the author's research and study (presented in Chap. 4), informed by Amram and Dryer (2008), who stated that 'spiritual intelligence is the ability to apply, manifest, and embody spiritual resources, values, and qualities to enhance daily functioning and wellbeing'.

2.3 Mental Health

'Vata', 'pitta' and 'kapha' are physical disorders and 'rajoguna' and 'tamoguna' are mental disorders.

Charaka Samhita (Sutra Sthan 1/56)

Because of individual, cultural and other variances, it is challenging to define mental health simply, since it is recognized that normality and mental health are highly contentious notions among psychologists. This section will first briefly examine what health means before going into the definition of mental health and its operational meaning. Ayurveda provides a very accurate definition of health ('swasthya'), describing it as the satisfaction of the 'atman' (soul or consciousness), the five senses, and the mind, in addition to the balance of the three 'doshas', thirteen 'agnis' (flames or metabolic fires), seven 'dhatus' (tissues), and waste product elimination processes:

समदोषः समाग्निश्च समधातुमलक्रियः।
Samdoshah samagnisch samdhatumalkriyah
प्रसन्नात्मेन्द्रियमनाः स्वस्थ इत्यभिधीयते।।
Prasannatmendriyamanah swasth ityabhidheeyate

(Shushruta Samhita, 15/41)

2.3.1 *What Is Health?*

The word 'health' in English derives from the old English word 'hale', which denotes wholeness, soundness or wellbeing. As the word's definition suggests, being healthy often refers to being well and disease-free. According to science, a living being's level of functional or metabolic efficiency is what is known as their health. Health was defined by the World Health Organization (1946) as 'a state of complete physical, mental, and social well-being and not merely the absence of disease or infirmity'. This notion of health was questioned due to some potential confusion it may have caused. The WHO modified the definition in the Ottawa Charter for Health Promotion in 1986 and said that health is: 'A resource for everyday life, not the objective of living. Health is a positive construct accenting social and personal resources, as well as physical capacities'. Although it (health) comprises both physical and mental health, the concept of health is typically conceived of as physiological health and wellbeing. As per *Merriam-Webster.com* (n.d.) health is: (1) the condition of being sound in body, mind or spirit; (2) a condition in which someone or something is thriving or doing well (wellbeing).

Health, alternatively, may be divided into the following three aspects (ACS Distance Education, n.d.):

1. *Emotional or Mental Health*: A person's overall condition of health and fitness is greatly influenced by their emotional health, also known as emotional intelligence. However, this influence is frequently undervalued.
2. *Structural Health*: The soundness of the body is structurally stable the bones, muscles, organs and so forth are physically in shape and not broken; performing the functions they must perform. Structural or physical health is often determined by considering someone's height/weight ratio, their body mass index, their resting heart rate and recovery time after exercise. Sometimes the second aspect structural health is replaced with the term 'spiritual health'.
3. *Chemical Health*: The chemicals in our body are right there are no lethal synthetic concoctions; the tissues are comprised of the fitting equalization of supplements or nutrients and so on.

In addition, the word 'wellness', is broadly defined as the quality or state of being healthy. Wellness is a state of optimum wellbeing that is oriented toward increasing an individual's potential. It is a deeply rooted procedure of moving towards improving our physical, intellectual, enthusiastic, social, spiritual and natural wellbeing. Wellness is most likely to mean a healthy balance of the mind, body and spirit that leads to an overall feeling of wellbeing. According to *AlleyDog.com* (n.d.):

> Wellness is a term that refers to an optimum level of health and fitness that allows an individual to function actively and fully over the full range of life activities; physical, emotional, spiritual, social, intellectual and environmental. Maintaining a state of wellness includes proper eating and sleeping habits, regular exercise, avoiding substance use/abuse, etc.

2.3.2 What Is Mental Health?

> सत्वं रजस्तम इति मानसाः स्युस्त्रयो गुणाः
> satvam rajastam iti maanasaah syustrayo gunaah,
> तेषां गुणानां साम्यं यक्त दाहुः स्वस्थलक्षणम्
> tesam gunanam saamyam yakt daahuh swasthlakshanam.
>
> 'Sattva', 'raja' and 'tama' are three mental traits. The balancing state of the three traits is the state of actual mental health.
>
> Mahabharata, Santiparva 16/13

When it comes to definitions of mental health, these usually refer to a state of psychological stability, or the absence of a psychological disorder. According to positive psychology or holistic perspectives, a person's capacity to enjoy life and strike a balance between daily activities and efforts to build resilience may be considered a sign of mental health. Good adaptability to a range of tasks and the expression of emotions are another two ways that mental health may be defined. According to the World Health Organization, mental health is 'a state of wellbeing within which the individual realizes his or her own abilities, can cope with the normal stresses of life, can work fruitfully and productively, and is in a position to make a contribution to his or her community'. According to the *Free Dictionary* (n.d.-b), mental health is 'a state of emotional and psychological wellbeing in which an individual is able to use his or her cognitive and emotional capabilities, function in society, and meet the ordinary demands of everyday life'. Furthermore, the dictionary defines mental health as 'a person's overall emotional and psychological condition'.

Mental health is generally the absence of any kind of mental disorder or disease. Mental health, in view of its dimensions, is easy to understand. Some psychiatrists, philosophers and anthropologists' views and studies on the concept of mental health and illness are as follows. Heinz (1994) described mental health on the basis of therapeutic goals shared among distinct psychotherapeutic approaches, and cautioned that flexibility of behaviour, empathy and self-efficacy ought to be the criteria of mental health that define functions required for a healthy living. Alienation is a core dimension of mental health. Jaeggi (2005) defined alienation as a form of unsuccessful interaction with the world, in which an individual expresses what feelings, wishes or goals he or she has. Alienation is then a description of a failed procedure rather than an assessment of the content or purpose implicated with the behaviour. Alienated behaviour can also consequently be characterized by inflexibility or an inability to express one's desires in a way that matches with one's preceding life narration and self-concepts. Mental health may then reasonably be described with the aid of all the resources that are known to positively affect disease outcomes. Fulford (1989) stressed the concept of 'action failure' as being the common thread. In both mental and physical illness, the patient experiences a lack of ability to function in daily living owing to physical or psychological difficulties. Fulford makes the clearest distinction between the words 'illness' and 'disease', seeing illness as essential to disease, with the illness being derived from the experience of an action failure, a failure in ordinary doing in daily life. The illness is then understood in terms of disease concepts applied to the features of the action failures that occur. Kleinman (1988) suggests that:

> Illness refers to the patient's perception, experience, expression, and pattern of coping with symptoms, while disease refers to the manner practitioners recast illness in terms of their theoretical models of pathology. Thus, a psychiatric diagnosis is an interpretation of a person's experience.

If we study the concept of '*normality*' deeply, then different meanings emerge, Sheldon J. Korchin (2004) collected all these meanings (citing various studies) in his book and gave the following explications:

- *Normality as health*: In this interpretation, which is common in both traditional medical-psychiatric terms and layman usage, normality simply means 'not sick.'
- *Normality as ideal*: This searches for a definition of what normality is in order to define it as an ideal or desired state. This class of viewpoints includes those that emphasize psychological development as a process of self-actualization, becoming a 'fully functioning person', or developing a 'mature personality'.
- *Averageness as normality*: The NPC (normal probability curve) measuring numbers led to the development of this point of view.

- *Normality as socially acceptable behaviour*: This theory contends that behaviour can only be judged in the context of its social environment. If it adheres to societal norms, it is regarded as normal; if not, it is viewed as deviant or abnormal.
- *Normality as process*: This attempts to define normality in terms of long-term processes rather than from a cross-sectional basis.

2.3.3 Models of Mental Health or Abnormality

There are various models of mental health or abnormality in psychology. Abnormality means behaviour, thinking processes or feelings deemed undesirable and so subject to regulation or change. Different theoretical orientations, tolerances for deviation, demarcations between the normal and abnormal, and labelling strategies result in divergent definitional standards. Subjective discomfort, incapacity or inefficiency, and deviance, particularly bizarre or reality-distorting deviance, are crucial requirements (Rodriguez, 2001).

- *Behavioural Model*: The development of maladaptive behaviours is explained by this model of abnormal behaviour using learning principles.
- *Biomedical Model*: This abnormality model investigates how biological, neurological, and medicinal elements lead to psychological problems.
- *Cognitive Model*: According to the cognitive viewpoint on psychopathology, faulty thinking, such as illogical or irrational thought patterns, result in abnormal behaviour.
- *Family Model*: Family members' psychopathologies have been linked to dysfunctional family communications and structures.
- *Humanistic-Existential Model*: According to this perspective, psychopathology results from emotions of emptiness, worthlessness, and alienation, from a lack of commitment, will and responsibility, as well as from a failure to develop and reach one's full potential.
- *Legal Model*: This model takes into account a person's inclination towards ineptitude or their incapacity to comprehend their legal obligations.
- *Psychodynamic Model*: The core tenet of the psychodynamic perspective is the significant role played by unconscious and internal psychological conflict in shaping human emotions, behaviour and the emergence of psychiatric diseases.
- *Sociocultural Models*: A sociocultural approach to abnormal psychology looks at how cultural variables influence what behaviour is classified as abnormal in various societies and how some types of psychological abnormality are increased by society norms.

2.3.4 The Operational Definition of Mental Health

Mental health has been chosen as a construct formed by Kumar and Thakur (1986) for the research and study (see Chap. 4) conducted by the author. Kumar and Thakur divided mental health into five dimensions:

1. *Egocentrism*: This is an indication of the concern for oneself and one's needs, feelings, opinions, and ideas. High scorers in this area might have trouble empathizing with or identifying with other people.
2. *Alienation*: The alienation dimension was created to show how much the response resembled hospitalized psychiatric patients. People with high scores in this area tend to be too circumspect, unusually sensitive and experience sensory distortions.
3. *Expression*: Expression is a sign of how socially interactive individuals are. A high score on this dimension implies a lack of social disclosure, inconsistent interactions in social settings and a sense of insecurity.
4. *Emotional Instability*: The emotional instability dimension reveals a person's level of happiness, nervousness, emotional labile, fear, anxiety and depression. A high score on this dimension suggests that the person needs psychological and psychiatric support and has major personality issues.
5. *Social nonconformity;* this reveals if the person is supporting or opposing the current social system. People with high scores on this dimension are likely to have higher social nonconformity.

2.4 Quality of Life

One of the most often used concepts; quality of life (QOL) has numerous definitions in philosophy, political science and health. Quality of life (QOL) reflects the general health of individuals and societies. It's frequently confused with the notion of a standard of living, which is largely based on income. Instead, good quality of life can be measured by factors like wealth and employment, as well as the built environment, one's physical and mental health, education, leisure activities and a sense of belonging (Geraldine et al., 2009). A wide, multifaceted notion, quality of life typically comprises subjective assessments of both positive and negative facets of life (WHOQOL, 1998). There are other dimensions of overall quality of life besides health that are equally essential, including jobs, housing, schools and the neighbourhood. Overall quality of life also includes important elements of culture, values and spirituality, which adds to the estimation's unpredictability. Moreover, QOL can be defined in a variety of ways, making it challenging to assess and include in scientific research. Any definition should be all-inclusive while allowing for the differentiation of specific components because sickness and its treatment affects people's biological integrity as well as their psychological, social and economic wellness. This makes it possible to assess how different disease states or therapies affect different facets of QoL overall or in specific circumstances.

The World Health Organization (n.d.) defined the term 'Quality of Life' as:

> an individual's perception of their position in life in the context of the culture and value systems in which they live and in relation to their goals, expectations, standards and concerns. It is a broad ranging concept affected in a complex way by the person's physical health, psychological state, personal beliefs, social relationships and their relationship to salient features of their environment.

Today quality of life is widely mentioned in several scientific fields. Quality of life in economics is studied as the standard of living; in sociology it is known as a subjective understanding and evaluation of wellbeing and in medical science the most common factor in quality of life study is the issue of health and illness. Health-related quality of life is the most discussed topic in quality-of-life research, which is discussed in the next section. Similar to other concepts like health and mental health, there is no single, clear-cut definition of quality of life.

Perhaps the concept of quality of life can best be understood as following interrelated domains discussed in the WHOQOL-BREF: physical health, psychological health, social relationships and environment.

1. *Physical Health*: This involves functional capacity, physical comfort, health promotion, and health maintenance.
2. *Psychological Health*: This includes mental health, social support, interpersonal dynamics, and cultural dynamics.
3. *Social Relationship*: This includes one's personal social system and the global societal system.
4. *Environment*: This includes socioeconomic status, transportation, assistive devices, safety, and aesthetics.

Some scholars further add these domains:

5. *Metaphysical Domain* (which includes self-esteem, self-determination, cognition, purpose, optimism and life satisfaction) and
6. *Spiritual Domains* (which includes prayer, worship, fellowship and meaning) in the scope of quality of life.

2.4.1 Health-Related Quality of Life (HRQOL)

The concept of health-related quality of life (HRQOL) came into existence because the term quality of life has various definitions depending on the subject and the place where the term is being used, such as in general it is taken as a standard of living, in economics as economic status, and in psychology and other behavioural sciences it is studied as a multidomain concept of overall wellbeing. With HRQOL, special attention is given to health and related concepts as indicators of life quality. Health-related QoL concepts include the physical, functional social and emotional well-being of the individual. The idea of HRQOL and its determinants have evolved since the 1980s to include those aspects of overall quality of life which are clearly shown to have an effect on health, either physical or mental (Selim et al., 2009). At an individual level, this encompasses perceptions of physical and mental health as well as their correlates, such as functional status, social support and socioeconomic status. It also includes health risks and conditions. The measurement of physical and mental decline, impaired role and social functioning, and HRQOL have historically been the focus of studies of quality of life in relation to health. These studies have traditionally been based on a pathology model of health and dependency. In other words, using the functionalism approach, it taps into how individuals carry out tasks that are crucial for the continuous operation of larger society. This approach for measuring has resulted in a negative focus, at the expense of the positive. For example, scales are constructed to measure levels of functional limitations, rather than balanced scales with equal measures of levels of ability (Bowling, 2001). According to a unique definitional approach, the gap between one's current level of health and functional status and one's aspirations is what constitutes HRQOL. This paradigm is based on social norms and peer comparisons. Although creative efforts are made to operationalize and quantify this gap, there is little evidence to support the model's content validity. The measurements of HRQOL all summarize people's assessments of their experiences with health and illness. This is a prevalent theme when discussing these metrics. A broader definition of health-related quality of life is whether ailment or impairment makes it difficult for a person to carry out daily activities.

2.4.2 The Operational Definition of Quality of Life

As per the WHOQOL Group (1994a, 1994b) 'quality of life is defined as individuals' perceptions of their position in life in the context of the culture and value systems in which they live and in relation to their goals, expectations, standards, and concerns'.

2.5 Early Adulthood

The author has carried out his research and study (see Chap. 4) on early adults, so this section explains the concepts of adulthood and early adulthood. The Latin verb *adolescere*, meaning 'to grow to maturity', is the same verb that gives the English word 'adult'. The word 'adult' is derived from the '*adultus*' which implies 'grown to full size and vigour' or 'matured'. Adults are thus people who have reached the culmination of their development and are ready to assume their status in society alongside other adults. The age at which a child becomes an adult, or the age of legal maturity, varies by culture. In the majority of older cultures, this age was reached when the child's puberty growth was complete, or nearly complete, and when the child's sex organs had sufficiently matured to be capable of procreation. Up until recently, children were not regarded as legal adults until they turned 21. Adulthood is now considered by law in the majority of nations to be reached at the age of 18.

Adulthood is currently by far the longest time period in the entire life cycle due to gradual increases in longevity. Certain physical and psychological changes take place over the lengthy span of adulthood at predictable intervals. Adulthood is traditionally divided based on the times at which these changes take place, along with the adjustment problems and cultural pressures and expectations that they give rise to. This is similar to how childhood and adolescence are long periods during which specific physical and psychological changes occur at predictable times. The years between our early twenties and old age and death can be thought of as adulthood. Precisely when a person becomes an adult is difficult to define. Cultural and other factors account for these challenges. Adulthood is reached in certain societies and cultures soon after puberty (Bledsoe & Cohen, 1993). Some believe that adulthood begins after high school, while others believe it doesn't begin until after college graduation. Young/early adulthood, middle adulthood and late adulthood are three major categories into which adulthood can be classified. These three stages are among the eight psychosocial life stages identified by Erikson. The sixth, seventh and eighth stages include crises occurring in these stages respectively: sixth stage: Early adulthood (intimacy versus isolation); seventh stage: Middle adulthood (generativity versus stagnation); and eighth stage: Late adulthood (ego integrity versus despair). Thus, the stages of adulthood may be generally divided into three broad phases: *early* (from approximately 18 to 40 years of age), *middle* (41 to 65) and *late* (66+).

References

ACS Distance Education. (n.d.). Retrieved April 8, 2020, from https://www.acs.edu.au/info/recreation-and-fitness/health/what-is-health.aspx

AlleyDog.com. (n.d.). Retrieved April 8, 2020, from https://www.alleydog.com/glossary/definition.php?term=Wellness

Amram, Y. (2007, August). *The seven dimensions of spiritual intelligence: An ecumenical grounded theory.* Paper presented at the 115th Annual Conference of the American Psychological Association.

Amram, Y., & Dryer, D. C. (2008, August). *The integrated spiritual intelligence scale (ISIS): Development and preliminary validation.* Paper presented at the 116th Annual Conference of the American Psychological Association.

Bledsoe, C. H., & Cohen, B. (1993). *Social dynamics of adolescent fertility in Sub-Saharan Africa.* National Academy Press.

Bowell, R. A. (2004). *The seven steps of spiritual intelligence.* Nicholas Brealey Publishing.

Bowling, A. (2001). *Measuring disease: A review of disease specific quality of life measurement scales* (2nd ed.). Open University Press.

Calvert, W. (2000). *The American Heritage Dictionary of Indo-European Roots* (2nd ed.). Houghton-Mifflin.

Ciccarelli, S. K., & Meyer, G. E. (2008). *Psychology.* Dorling Kindersley Pvt. Ltd.

Dhar, N., Datta, U., & Nandan, D. (2008). Importance of spiritual health in public health systems of India. *Health and Population—Perspectives and Issues, 31(3)*, 204–211.

Dictionary.com. (n.d.). Retrieved April 9, 2020, from http://dictionary.reference.com/browse/spirituality?s=t

Emmons, R. (1999). *The psychology of ultimate concerns: Motivation and spirituality in personality.* Guilford.

Emmons, R. (2000). Spirituality and intelligence: Problems and prospects. *International Journal for the Psychology of Religion, 10*(1), 57–64.

Fulford, K. W. M. (1989). *Moral theory and medical practice.* Cambridge University Press.

Geraldine, P., Gregory, D., & Johnston, R. (2009). *Quality of life. Dictionary of human geography* (5th ed.). Wiley-Blackwell.

Hassed, C. S. (2000). Depression: Dispirited or spiritually deprived? *Medical Journal of Australia, 173*(10), 545–547.

Heinz, A. (1994). *Der Begriff psychischer Gesundheit* (Unpublished master's thesis). Freie Universität Berlin.

Humphreys, J. (2000). Spirituality and distress in sheltered battered women. *Journal of Nursing Scholarship, 32*(3), 273–278.

Jaeggi, R. (2005). *Entfremdung. Zur Aktualität eines sozialphilosophischen Problems.* Campus Verlag.

Kleinman, A. (1988). *Rethinking psychiatry: From cultural category to personal experience.* Free Press.

Korchin, S. J. (2004). *Modern clinical psychology.* Basic Books, Reprinted by CBS Publishers.

Kumar, A., & Thakur, G. P. (1986). *Mithila Mental Health Status Inventory (MMHSI).* Ganga Saran and Grand Sons.

Lama, D. (1999). *Ethics for the New Millennium.* Riverhead Books.

Levin, M. (2000). *Spiritual intelligence: Awakening the power of your spirituality and intuition.* Hodder and Stoughton.

Living Words of Wisdom. (n.d.). Retrieved April 9, 2020, from http://www.livingwordsofwisdom.com/definition-of-spirituality.html

McSherry, W. (2000). Education issues surrounding the teaching of spirituality. *Nursing Standard, 14*(42), 40–43.

Merriam-Webster.com. (n.d.). Retrieved April 8, 2020, from https://www.merriam-webster.com/dictionary/health

Nasel, D. D. (2004). *Spiritual orientation in relation to spiritual intelligence: A new consideration of traditional Christianity and New Age/individualistic spirituality* (Doctoral Dissertation). University of South Australia.

Oldnall, A. (1996). A critical analysis of nursing: Meeting the spiritual needs of patients. *Journal of Advanced Nursing, 23*(1), 138–144.

Order of Time.com. (n.d.). Retrieved April 9, 2020, from http://www.theorderoftime.com/spiritual/spiritualessence.html#The%20definition%20of%20spirituality

Oxford Dictionaries. (n.d.-a). Retrieved April 9, 2020, from http://www.oxforddictionaries.com/definition/english/spirit?q=spirit

Oxford Dictionaries. (n.d.-b). Retrieved April 9, 2020, from https://www.lexico.com/definition/religious

Oxford Dictionaries. (n.d.-c). Retrieved April 9, 2020, from https://www.lexico.com/definition/religion

Rodriguez, J. (2001). *Psychology and mental health.* Salem Press.

Selim, A. J., Rogers, W., Fleishman, J. A., Qian, S. X., Fincke, B. G., Rothendler, J. A., & Kazis, L. E. (2009). Updated US population standard for the Veterans RAND 12-item Health Survey (VR-12). *Quality of Life Research, 18*(1), 43–52.

Sheldrake, P. (2007). *A brief history of spirituality.* Blackwell.

The Free Dictionary. (n.d.-a). Retrieved April 9, 2020, from http://www.thefreedictionary.com/spirituality

The Free Dictionary (n.d.-b). Retrieved April 9, 2020, from https://www.thefreedictionary.com/Mental+health

Tisdell, E. J. (2003). *Exploring spirituality and culture in adult and higher education.* Jossey-Bass.

Vaughan, F. (2002). What is spiritual intelligence?. *Journal of Humanistic Psychology, 42*(2), 16–33.

Waaijman, K. (2002). *Spirituality: Forms, foundations, methods.* Peeters.

WHOQOL. (1998). The World Health Organization Quality of Life assessment (WHOQOL). Development and psychometric properties. *Social Science & Medicine, 46*, 1569–1585.

WHOQOL Group. (1994a). Development of the WHOQOL: Rationale and current status. *International Journal of Mental Health, 23*(3), 24–56.

WHOQOL Group. (1994b). The development of the World Health Organization Quality of Life assessment instrument (the WHOQOL). In J. Orley & W. Kuyken (Eds.), *Quality of life assessment: International perspectives*. Springer Verlag.

Wigglesworth, C. (2006). Why spiritual intelligence is essential to mature leadership. *Integral Leadership Review, 6*, 14–15.

Wigglesworth, C. (2011). *Integral theory (also called AQAL theory) and its relationship to spiritual intelligence and the SQi assessment.* Deep Change.

Wolman, R. (2001). *Thinking with your soul: Spiritual intelligence and why it matters.* Harmony.

World Health Organization. (1946). *WHO definition of health.* Preamble to the Constitution of the World Health Organization as adopted by the International Health Conference.

World Health Organization. (n.d.). Retrieved April 8, 2020, from https://www.who.int/healthinfo/survey/whoqol-qualityoflife/en/

Zohar, D., & Marshall, I. (2000). *Spiritual intelligence: The ultimate intelligence.* Bloomsbury.

Zohar, D., & Marshall, I. (2004). *Spiritual capital: Wealth we can live by.* Berrett-Koehler Publishers.

Chapter 3
The Relationship of Spirituality with Mental Health and Quality of Life: A Review

It is clear to see that the challenge of mental illness is escalating rapidly. According to data from the World Health Organization, roughly half of the world's population suffers from a mental disease that affects their capacity to form relationships, to function in daily life, and their self-esteem (Storrie et al., 2010). This reveals adverse consequences for two of the crucial requirements for quality of life and mental health. Spirituality in the form of spiritual intelligence and other related dimensions are new concepts in the affected area, so this study represents a crucial step in the comprehension of the impact of spirituality on early adults' mental health and quality of life. This study, like several earlier ones, will support the worth and significance of spiritual intelligence in terms of mental health and overall quality of life. Here is an illustration of how spiritual intelligence might manifest in our day-to-day lives: We would feel unaffected whether someone compliments the clothes we are wearing, offends us in any manner, or makes a derogatory remark about how we appear, because we understand that our true beauty is found in our nature and character. In past research, the concepts of spirituality and religiosity were often taken as the same construct. Currently, spirituality in modern studies has come to be seen as a type of intelligence, that is, the ultimate intelligence or spiritual intelligence (SQ). Because the study and research described in Chapter 4 are in accord with this modern construct of spiritual intelligence, it strengthens the value of the study, which will be new in the Indian scenario with this developed construct. This chapter will offer a brief review of some past studies on 'spirituality and mental health', 'spirituality and quality of life', and other constructs affecting spirituality, mental health and quality of life, conducted both in India and worldwide, to get a broader view of all these constructs.

N. Pant, *Spirituality, Mental Health and Quality of Life*,
https://doi.org/10.1007/978-981-99-2703-6_3

3.1 Spirituality and Mental Health

A meta-analysis of religiosity and mental health was done by Bergin (1983). The presumption that religiosity is inherently connected with psychopathology was refuted in a meta-analysis of 24 studies on the correlation between religiosity and personality, but Bergin also found only marginally favourable correlates of religion. Finally, researchers suggested that *religion reflects a multifaceted phenomenon with both positive and negative aspects.* Religious faith and spirituality are examined by Pardini et al. (2000) to ascertain the advantages for mental health. They looked at the relationship between spirituality, religious faith and the outcomes in terms of mental health in 236 people who were recovering from substance abuse. They discovered that *although people in recovery frequently report having strong religious beliefs and affiliations, they prefer to consider themselves as being more spiritual than religious.* ***The findings also showed that among those in recovery, higher levels of spirituality and religious faith were linked to a more optimistic outlook on life, stronger feelings of social support, stronger stress resilience, and lower levels of anxiety.*** To determine the relationships between spirituality and religion and acute cardiovascular reactions, Lawler and Younger (2002) conducted research. In their study, physical symptoms of disease, stress and psychological mood were examined in a community sample of adults. They discovered that *resting diastolic and mean arterial pressure were related to religiousness, frequency of worship attendance, and affiliation with a particular religion.* ***There was a relationship between spirituality and disease symptoms. Further spirituality was found to be related with medicine use, stress, and negative moods. A deeper sense of purpose and meaning in life is linked to greater resilience and resistance to stress-related illness, and engaging in spirituality and organised religion may be a way to achieve this.*** In a population with chronic pain, Rippentrop et al. (2005) looked into the relationships between spirituality/religion, physical and mental health, and pain. They found that the religious and spiritual beliefs of pain patients differ from those of the general public (e.g., pain patients feel less desire to reduce pain and feel more abandoned by God). ***Significant relations between elements of religion/spirituality and physical and mental health were found by using hierarchical multiple regression analysis.*** *The results of private religious activity (such as prayer, meditation, and the consumption of religious media) were inversely correlated with those of physical health outcomes, suggesting that people with worse physical health were more likely to engage in private religious activity, possibly as a coping mechanism.* ***In addition to self-ratings of religious/spiritual intensity, everyday spiritual experiences, negative religious coping, and forgiveness all strongly predicted mental health status.*** *Religion and spirituality have little bearing on the severity of pain or how much it interferes with daily life.* In a stratified, random sample of college students, Zullig et al. (2006) investigated the mediating effect of self-reported health between perceived spirituality, religiosity and life satisfaction while controlling for gender. And found ***Students who identify as spiritual or religious are more likely to report higher levels of self-perceived health, and life satisfaction is likely to be influenced by both men's and women's levels of***

self-perceived health. *The findings suggest that different reported health statuses, both physical and mental, are associated to different levels of life satisfaction and that involvement in religion and spirituality may have an impact on life satisfaction.* Nagel and Sgoutas-Emch (2007) used measures of both spirituality and religion in a study on college students in the United States to investigate if the same pattern of relationships observed previously was visible in a sample of healthy college students. *The results found that* ***the people who scored higher on the spirituality measurement were more active and had different health beliefs from people who did not***. Faribors et al. (2010) studied the relationship between spiritual intelligence and happiness among nurses in Iran. *The findings revealed* ***a significant link between spiritual intelligence and happiness***. *Spiritual intelligence and happiness were significantly related with demographic traits.* Babanazari et al. (2012) studied spiritual intelligence and happiness among adolescents at high school. According to the study's findings, *spiritual intelligence and happiness are significantly correlated. According to the findings of the regression analysis, happiness was significantly predicted by awareness sensing, mystery sensing, value sensing, and community sensing.* A descriptive and correlational study on the occupational stress and spiritual intelligence of members of the National Company of Oil Products was conducted by Ahmadian et al. (2013). And found ***a relationship between spiritual intelligence and occupational stress among employees of the company***. Do existential factors mediate between the religious-spiritual aspects of functionality and psychological wellbeing? This question was the focus of Wnuk and Marcinkowski's (2014) research. They observed the *meaning of life and hope to mediate between spiritual experiences and life satisfaction as well as between spiritual experiences and positive aspects. Negative effects were not linked to spiritual experiences. Hope and the meaning of life both anticipated negative effect.* ***Meaning of life and hope were discovered to be important factors in the religion-wellbeing link and associated to favourable psychological outcomes, such as increased life satisfaction and positive effects as well as diminished negative effects***. In their study, Alihosseini et al. (2014) examined the relation between youths' happiness and spiritual intelligence. According to the Pearson correlation results, ***inner peace, spiritual experiences, forgiveness, and self-recognition—all the components (of spiritual intelligence)—have positive and significant relationship with happiness.*** *The independent t-test results also revealed a significant difference between male and female students in the link between spiritual intelligence and happiness, with both variables being higher in female students.*

Research studies in India: In order to study predicting effects on adolescents' mental health, Singh et al. (2010) looked at spiritual intelligence, altruism, school environment and academic achievement. Multiple correlation and regression analyses of the data showed that the ***type of school, spiritual intelligence, altruism, rejection (a dimension of the school environment) and control (a dimension of the school environment) were the important predictors of mental health***. *Additionally, factors like gender, place of residence, creative stimulation, acceptance, permissiveness and academic success did not significantly predict mental health.* Dar et al.

(2011) looked into the relationship between male police officers' psychological wellbeing and their emotional intelligence. According to the findings, male police officers are in a good position in terms of their emotional intelligence and psychological wellbeing. *Additionally, a strong positive association between emotional intelligence and psychological wellbeing was discovered.* Religiosity was examined in relation to anxiety and spirituality by Khan et al. (2014). Two age groups participated in the study: those between the ages of 20 and 40 and those between the ages of 60 and 80. They found:

1. No association between overall spirituality and anxiety, between participants of different ages, but a strong positive relationship between religiosity and anxiety.
2. On the religiosity scale, there was no noticeable difference between the older and younger age groups.
3. On the spirituality scale, there was a noticeable difference between the two groups: people aged 55–70 were determined to be highly spiritual.
4. On the anxiety scale, there was once more a significant difference between the two groups; the age range of 55–70 was shown to be much more anxious than the other group due to the age group's increased reliability with regard to religious views.
5. On the religious aspect and anxiety, there was a significant mean difference between the male and female participants. It was shown that female participants were more anxious and religious than the male ones.
6. On the spiritual aspect, there were no differences between the male and female groups.

Pant and Srivastava (2014) further studied the effect of spiritual intelligence on mental health and quality of life among college students, exploring any relationships among these three variables. Findings of the study revealed that ***there is a significant correlation between spiritual intelligence and quality of life, as well as between spiritual intelligence and mental health.*** *Lastly, they found a significant correlation between mental health and quality of life.* In a recent study done by Pant and Srivastava (2019) to find out the impact of spiritual intelligence, gender and educational background on mental health among college students, they found that ***students studying in the arts have a significant relationship between spiritual intelligence and mental health****, and there is a significant relationship between spiritual intelligence and mental health for both male and female arts students separately.* ***Students studying science have a significant relationship between spiritual intelligence and mental health****, and there is a significant relationship between spiritual intelligence and mental health among male and female science students separately.*

3.2 Spirituality and Quality of Life

There are a number of past studies on spiritual intelligence and quality of life Gioiella et al. (1998) examined the spirituality and quality of life of patients with gynecologic cancers and advised that taking patients' spiritual wellbeing into account in healthcare assessments could help identify their needs and coping mechanisms. They found that ***other than ovarian cancer, patients with gynecologic cancers reported higher QOL and greater levels of spiritual, existential, and religious wellbeing***. *In comparison to younger patients, older patients consistently reported higher levels of spiritual wellbeing and QOL. Patients who were married on average reported more spiritual wellbeing than those who were not married (never married or separated). Catholic patients outperformed other patients in terms of both Functional Living Index: Cancer (FLIC) scores and levels of spiritual and religious wellbeing.* Typically, health researchers do not consider a patient's spiritual health when assessing their needs. This study's findings suggest that routine patient assessment and intervention should take spirituality into account. Clinical interventions that would raise a patient's spiritual awareness and comfort level in relation to a personal viewpoint on death may aid in reducing the patient's psychosocial distress. *They finally concluded, religion and spirituality are positively related with both physical and mental health, despite the medical establishment's bias to the contrary, and may be especially important to patients who are terminally ill.* Further Walker and Dixon (2002) carried out a study of the spirituality and academic performance of African American college students, *and found that African Americans participate in religion and have higher degrees of spiritual belief than do European Americans. They discovered through correlation studies that both groups' spiritual beliefs and participation in religion were positively associated with academic performance; however, the nature of the association varied. For African Americans, participation and beliefs were important, whereas for European Americans, participation was important.* Further, Koenig (2004) conducted research on spirituality, wellness and quality of life, and ***uncovered the link between spirituality and general improvements in mental health, well-being and quality of life***. A meta-analysis of the relationship between spirituality and quality of life was carried out by Sawatzky et al. (2005). They discovered that a random effects model of the bivariate correlation between spirituality and quality of life produced a moderate effect size, supporting the study's theoretical framework in which spirituality is shown as a distinct idea that is related to quality of life. *The range in estimates of the degree of the association was linked to operational definitions of spirituality and quality of life, according to their further regression results.* In a study, Abdel-Khalek (2010) examined the religiousness, subjective well-being, and quality of life among Muslim college students, and concluded that, *based on the considerable and favourable correlations between quality of life, spiritual wellbein, and religiosity in this sample of Muslim college students, religiosity may be considered as a salient component of and a contributing factor to quality of life.* Ahmadi et al. (2012) examined the relationship between life quality and spiritual intelligence and accepting responsibility. According to their research findings, *transcendental* *awareness, one of the subscales of spiritual intelligence, accounts for a greater proportion of the life quality of the students when it comes to explaining that quality; consequently, as transcendental awareness increases, so does the influence it has on life quality. Additionally, among the components of taking responsibility, feeling responsibility contributes more to understanding the students' quality of life, such that when feeling responsibility rises, so does quality of life. Additionally, various subscales of taking responsibility, such as feeling secure, self-esteem, belongingness, and taking responsibility, have a favorable impact on the students' quality of life.* In a study on the importance of spiritual intelligence in predicting the quality of life of university students, Bolghan-Abadi et al. (2014) conducted research. The purpose of the study was to look at the function that spiritual intelligence plays in predicting the quality of life of Quchan University students. The results of the study showed that ***quality of life can be well predicted by spiritual intelligence.***

Research studies in India: Quality of life in the area of HIV/AIDS was researched by Basavaraj et al. (2010). The importance and complexity of physical, psychological and social aspects as predictors of health-related quality of life in HIV-infected people were underlined in this review. Through analysis of the available data, they proposed that *key predictors of QOL in this population were physical symptoms, antiretroviral therapy, psychological wellbeing, social support networks, coping mechanisms, spiritual wellbeing*, and mental comorbidities. As a result, a major concern for HIV-positive individuals is how HIV infection affects QOL characteristics like physical and emotional wellbeing, social supports and life roles. Singh and Sinha (2013) conducted research to determine the effect of spiritual intelligence on the QOL of government organization executives. A sample of 303 executives was chosen for this study, with a good representation at the junior, middle and senior levels. Three findings were:

1. *It was discovered that officers in older age ranges had, on average, higher SQ than the younger group, though not always.*
2. *Both male and female officers' SQ was reported to be equivalent, with the men's being just a little bit higher.*
3. *Most of the conditions when SQ was high, QOL was also higher.*

Kaur and Kaur (2014) investigated the impact of organizational spirituality on job satisfaction, workplace stress and quality of life. According to the findings, employees who have *high organizational spirituality levels are more satisfied with their jobs, have better work-life balance, and experience less occupational stress.* The study's conclusions also emphasized the need for promoting spiritual values in the workplace because doing so results in improved problem-solving abilities, less conflict, and greater job satisfaction, all of which contribute to the success of the organization. Pant and Srivastava (2015) further studied spiritual intelligence, gender and educational background as related to the quality of life of college students, *and found that,* ***among arts students, there was a considerable association between spiritual intelligence and quality of life****; this relationship was present for both male and female arts students separately.* ***In science students, there was a considerable association between spiritual intelligence and quality of life****; this relationship was* *present for both male and female science students.* Furthermore, in terms of quality of life, there was no noticeable difference between male and female students. Further, in terms of quality of life, there was no noticeable difference between students studying the arts or sciences.

3.3 Spirituality, Gender and Other Correlates

If we take a further look at some past studies on spiritual intelligence, gender and other correlates, we find various studies. A study by Deaux and Taynor (1973), on male and female college students, evaluated competence and intellect. They discovered that highly competent males received higher ratings than similarly qualified females, whereas low-competence males received lower ratings than comparable females. Petrides and Furnham (2000) examined gender differences in trait emotional intelligence that was both measured and self-reported. It was discovered that females exceeded males on the trait emotional intelligence measure of social skills. However, it was shown that males believed they had higher emotional intelligence than females when the 15 aspects of self-estimated emotional intelligence were integrated into a single scale and the participants' measured trait emotional intelligence scores were held constant. The majority of the substantial and positive relationships between measured and self-estimated scores show that persons have some awareness of their emotional intelligence. Males typically had larger correlations between measured and self-estimated scores than females, and a *regression analysis showed that self-reported emotional intelligence was significantly predicted by gender.* Are women more religious than men? An analysis was done by Loewenthal et al. (2002) addressing this very question. Additionally, gender variations in religious practices across various religious groups in the UK, was studied. Women reported being substantially less involved in their religion than men, although this effect was only shown in non-Christian communities. They also concluded that *whether women or men are more religious depends on their culture and the testing technique.* In a further study, African American college students' racial identities and religion preferences were examined by Sanchez and Carter (2005). Through multiple regression analyses they found that *the religious orientation was predicted by attitudes toward racial identity. The relationships between these variables were considerably influenced by gender as well.* Emotional intelligence and gender were examined by Naghavi and Redzuan (2011). They evaluated empirical studies that focused on how gender and emotional intelligence relate to one another. The study demonstrated a significant relationship between emotional intelligence and gender disparities. They found *girls to be higher than boys in terms of emotional intelligence,* whereas boys having high emotional intelligence was observed to be better in predicting achievement.

Research studies in India: Gender variations in emotional intelligence among Chandigarh (India)'s adolescent boys and girls were examined by Katyal and Awasthi (2005). In the results *emotional intelligence scores for girls were found to be higher than those for boys. Nevertheless, the disparities were significant at just the 0.10* *level.* Kaur et al. (2012) investigated the importance of psychology and spirituality in emotional intelligence. This study looked at emotional intelligence in relation to gender, spiritual quotient and various academic subjects of study. It was found that *the emotional intelligence of psychology students was higher than that of the other two categories. Emotional intelligence was significantly impacted by different spiritual quotient levels, but gender differences were not statistically significant.* In a further study, Khan and Singh (2013) looked at how gender influenced teachers' gratitude, spirituality and forgiveness. They observed *significant gender differences among male and female teachers in terms of gratitude, spirituality and forgiveness. Male teachers were found to be higher than the females in gratitude, and female teachers were found to be higher than males in terms of spirituality and forgiveness.* Saxena and Jain (2013) examined undergraduate students' social intelligence in regard to their gender and academic stream. The results of the gender and stream analyses showed that *female students had higher levels of social intelligence than male students, and that students in the arts had higher levels of social intelligence than students in other disciplines.*

3.4 Mental Health, Gender and Other Correlates

In an investigation of some past studies on mental health, gender and other correlates, the following studies are relevant. The question: How does gender affect stress, self-esteem and mental health? was explored by Zuckerman (1989). In most areas of life, men and women reported similar levels of stress, although women reported higher levels of stress related to family relationships and worries about their mental health. The men reported that they become more active in response to stress, but the women said they experienced more symptoms of depression and anxiety and were more prone to communicate their anger and feelings. Stress levels and responses were linked to self-esteem, interpersonal self-confidence and self-concepts in both men and women. The results indicated that *more persuasively than variations in stress, sex differences in self-concept can account for sex differences in dysfunctional reactivity to stress.* The effects of gender and a family history of alcoholism were examined in Kushner and Sher's (1993) study on the comorbidity of alcohol and anxiety disorders among college students. They found that individuals with an anxiety diagnosis had a considerably higher percentage of respondents with an alcohol diagnosis. Male respondents and those with a family history of alcoholism had a base rate of alcohol disorder that was much higher than that of other individuals. However, these characteristics did not interact with (i.e., moderate) comorbidity risk; that is, they did not impact the proportionate increase in risk for an alcohol disorder associated with the presence of an anxiety disorder. They focused on topics important to recognizing and differentiating between interaction effects and base-rate effects in comorbidity research while presenting these results. In a further study, the gender differences in many aspects of psychological wellbeing were researched by Roothman et al. (2003). There was a statistically significant gender difference with small to medium practical implications. *On measures of physical self-concept, automatic thoughts (positive), constructive thinking, cognitive flexibility, overall self-concept, and fortitude, males performed better than females. While females performed better in terms of affect expression, physical symptoms, and religious wellbeing.* On the social components of self-concept and fortitude as well as on affect balance, emotional intelligence, self-efficacy and sense of coherence, there were no significant gender differences. In a another study on unemployment and mental health, Artazcoz et al. (2004) explored the interactions between gender, family responsibilities and socioeconomic class. They looked at how unemployment affects people differently depending on their gender and evaluated whether these impacts are related to interactions between social class, family roles and gender. *Men's mental health was impacted by unemployment more than women's was.* Effects on gender varied depending on social class and familial responsibilities. In their study, Brabete and Sánchez-López (2012) explored how gender affects people's health. Data was on a sample of Romanians who reside in Spain. The findings demonstrated *a strong relationship between gender socialisation and health-related behaviours.* Given that up to 50% of the variation in mortality and morbidity data can be attributed to healthy behaviour, they attest to the multiple factors influencing health and the multifaceted nature of gender. For every feminine or masculine gender standard, there are dangers or particular costs. They also observed that in order to accurately envision norms as valuable predictors of health behaviours in various groups of women and men, cultural variances in femininity and masculinity had to be taken into account.

Research studies in India: College students' attitudes and expectancies towards alcohol were examined by Kirmani and Suman (2010) to understand any evident gender disparities. The findings showed that *compared to girls, boys experienced higher levels of psychological distress and a more positive attitude toward alcohol. In addition, boys believed that drinking may result in good outcomes, but girls believed that drinking could result in bad things.* In a further study, Gupta and Kumar (2010) examined how college students' emotional intelligence and self-efficacy related to their mental health. According to the findings, *self-efficacy and emotional intelligence are positively associated with mental health. Additionally, it was found that male students outperformed female students in terms of self-efficacy, emotional intelligence, and mental health.* In another study college students' stress levels and coping skills were examined by Kumar and Bhukar (2013). The purpose of this study was to look into the stress levels and coping strategies of professional students studying engineering and physical education. The results of a two-way analysis of variance revealed that *girls in their profession experienced significantly more stress than boys due to all of the stressors. Boys in each field had a stronger coping strategy than girls, while girls in physical education had a higher coping strategy than both boys and girls in engineering. Finally, it is determined that students in physical education had stronger coping skills than those in engineering.* In another study in Rayalaseema Zone, Andhra Pradesh, India, Rao and Swathi (2013) investigated the mental health condition of degree college lecturers depending on gender and teaching experience. The study's findings indicated that *there were notable differences between professors who were male or female. In comparison to male lecturers,* *female had better mental health. For both genders, lecturers with more than ten years of experience were better at maintaining mental health than those with less than ten.* Joshi and Garg (2013) examined academicis' mental health in relation to their term of service. Additionally, data were gathered from academic institutions Dehradun, Uttarakhand, India. This study's mean and F ratio *results showed a considerable difference in the mental health of the two genders. Additionally, the study found a significant difference between service lengths of more than ten years and less than five years.* Nisa (2013) investigated how personality traits and familial issues affected college students' mental health. Additionally, a sample was obtained from the Albarkaat Public School in Aligarh, and the Aligarh Muslim University. *Among all personality traits, extraversion was found to be a major predictor of positive self-evaluation, according to the results of a multiple regression analysis. Openness also appeared as a strong predictor of reality perception and agreeableness for personality integration. Similarly, the environmental competence factor of students' mental health is highly predicted by extraversion and conscientiousness. However, only two aspects of mental health, positive self-evaluation and environmental competence, were predicted by familial issues.* Additionally, the results of the t-test showed that *the extraversion, openness, and agreeableness personality traits differ considerably between the male and female student groups. The integration of the personality and environmental competence elements of mental health is another area where they considerably vary. Compared to their male counterparts, female college students performed better on tests measuring environmental competence, one of the dimensions of mental health.* However, there was no gender difference detected in family difficulties. In another study, college students' stress levels and coping mechanisms in regard to their academic performance were examined by Ashwini and Barre (2014). The results showed that there is a big variation in how much stress students undergo. *The adjustment areas of students in the arts and sciences differ significantly. The academic performance of boys and girls differs significantly. The academic performance of the arts and sciences differs significantly.* Boys and girls in the arts and sciences, however, did not demonstrate any noticeable gender differences. Sharma (2014) investigated how gender and stream affected adolescents' depression. The findings showed that stream and gender had a significant interaction effect on adolescents' depression levels. Both were interdependent in terms of how they affected the students' depression scores. Additionally, differences in depression were found in terms of gender and stream. *Girls scored higher on depression than boys did, while arts students scored higher on depression than science and business students. Furthermore, it was noted that boys from the science, arts and commerce streams did not significantly differ on depression; however girls from these same streams did, with arts girls favouring it. There were no notable gender discrepancies in the science and commerce streams. However, in the arts stream, there were noticeable gender disparities on depression, with more girls than boys. The study's findings showed that gender and stream had a distinct impact on adolescent depression levels.*

3.5 Quality of Life, Gender and Other Correlates

If we take a further look at some past studies on quality of life and gender and other correlates, the following studies are found to be relevant. Age, gender and quality of life were all variables in a study by Mercier et al. (1998). The impact of age and gender on the subjective quality of life of people with severe and persistent mental illness is discussed in this study. Results revealed that there was *no difference in life quality between men and women; nevertheless, age was systematically associated with life satisfaction, with older individuals reporting higher levels of life satisfaction than their younger counterparts. Fewer older, happier respondents reported fears, a desire for change, or future plans in their responses to the open-ended questions.* In another study the relationship between quality of life and post-traumatic stress disorder (PTSD) in male and female veterans was examined by Schnurr and Lunney (2008). They discovered that a four-factor structure for the Quality of Life Inventory offered the greatest fit for both groups, using confirmatory factor analysis. *Overall, both men and women had poor quality of life; they did not differ significantly in either quality of life or the relationship between PTSD and quality of life; the few statistically significant differences were low and clinically insignificant. Numbing was uniquely linked to a lower quality of life for both men and women.* Akinyemi and Aransiola (2010) conducted research on the gender perspectives of elderly people in south-western Nigeria while they self-assessed their quality of life. *They discovered that, on some of the metrics, older women performed better than males. Additionally, women were more likely than their spouses to be able to cope on their own. Results from males with a living spouse revealed that, in comparison to the male, the majority of the spouses (females) were more likely to require assistance for routine daily activities. Men reported having superior sexual, psychological, and physical health levels. The study came to the conclusion that because of the various problems and responsibilities faced by men, measures of quality of life were likely to favour elderly women over elderly men.* Craciun (2013) investigated how gender, self-criticism and coping strategies relate to quality of life. In total, 228 psychology and law students were examined. The *findings revealed significant disparities in the choice of coping strategies between males and females. Additionally, the task-oriented, emotion-focused, gender-specific and self-critical factors of coping methods were found to be strongly associated to quality of life.* In a further research King Khalid University (Mohail Assermore) students' health-related quality of life was the subject of a study done by Megahed (2014). Results showed that the study sample had lower mean scores across the majority of eight health dimensions. The study sample's sex, kind of education and eight health dimensions varied significantly. *The study's findings showed that the study sample had a lower health-related quality of life; female students scored lower than male students.*

Research studies in India: Life satisfaction among professional and non-professional students in India was investigated by Shirazi and Khan (2013). No statistically significant differences were found between the mean scores of professional students' life satisfaction when residence and gender were taken into account.

Consideration of domicile and gender revealed a substantial variation in the mean life satisfaction scores of nonprofessional students. The findings indicate that, when compared to female students, male students have higher mean life satisfaction scores. In a study, Kumar (2014) examined the level of life satisfaction among teachers in primary, middle, and secondary schools in the district of Kathua. The results showed that there was no noticeable difference in the life satisfaction of teachers who were male and female (on a gender basis). *The level of life satisfaction differed significantly among teachers working in various sorts of institutions (i.e., government. and private). Compared to teachers working in private schools, those working in government schools reported higher levels of satisfaction.* Additionally, there was no noticeable difference in interaction between gender (male and female), and government. and private institution type.

3.6 Conclusion

As it has been seen, there is little doubt that there are ample shreds of evidence showing a positive relationship between spirituality/religiosity and mental health/ quality of life. According to a study by Elmer et al. (2003), spirituality helps people live longer and suffer less from diseases. Spiritually inclined people appear to respond to assistance better after suffering an accident, endure trauma better, and have less depression (Emmons, 2000; MacDonald & Friedman, 2002). Trott's (1996) study also indicated positive correlations between spiritual wellbeing and general self-efficacy. On the basis of this review analysis, it could be concluded that spirituality, including religiosity, is positively correlated to mental health and quality of life. Spirituality and religiosity play a predicting and significant role in determining mental health and quality of life. And gender, age, educational stream and socioeconomic status play a significant determining role in terms of spirituality, mental health and quality of life. Whether the present trend is moving towards new concepts in spirituality, such as spiritual intelligence, spiritual wellbeing and so forth, yet we still need more scientific and well-developed constructs to find out better outcomes in the field of mental health and quality of life.

References

Abdel-Khalek, A. M. (2010). Quality of life, subjective well-being, and religiosity in Muslim college students. *Quality of Life Research, 19*(8), 1133–1143.

Ahmadi, A., Ahghar, G., & Abedi, M. R. (2012). The relationship between spiritual intelligence and taking responsibility with life quality. *European Online Journal of Natural and Social Sciences, 2*(3), 391–400.

Ahmadian, E., Hakimzadeh, A., & Kordestani, S. (2013). Job stress and spiritual intelligence: A case study. *World Applied Sciences Journal, 22*(11), 1667–1676.

Akinyemi, A., & Aransiola, J. (2010). Gender perspectives in self-assessment of quality of life of the elderly in south-western Nigeria. *Journal of Comparative Research in Anthropology and Sociology, 1*(1), 107–120.

Alihosseini, F., Rangan, U., Alihosseini, A., & Hajmohammadi, F. (2014). A study of the relationship between spiritual intelligence and its components with happiness in youths. *The International Journal of Humanities & Social Studies, 2*(6), 56–60.

Artazcoz, L., Benach, J., Borrell, C., & Cortès, I. (2004). Unemployment and mental health: Understanding the interactions among gender, family roles, and social class. *American Journal of Public Health: January, 94*(1), 82–88.

Ashwini, R., & Barre, V. P. (2014). Stress and adjustment among college students in relation to their academic performance. *Indian Journal of Health and Wellbeing, 5*(3), 288–292.

Babanazari, L., Askari, P., & Honarmand, M. M. (2012). Spiritual intelligence and happiness for adolescents in high school. *Life Science Journal, 9*(3), 2296–2299.

Basavaraj, K. H., Navya, M. A., & Rashmi, R. (2010). Quality of life in HIV/AIDS. *Indian Journal of Sexually Transmitted Diseases and AIDS, 31*(2), 75–80.

Bergin, A. E. (1983). Religiosity and mental health: A critical re-evaluation and meta-analysis. *Professional Psychology: Research and Practice, 14*(2), 170–184.

Bolghan-Abadi, M., Ghofrani, F., & Abde-Khodaei, M. S. (2014). Study of the spiritual intelligence role in predicting university students' quality of life. *Journal of Religion and Health, 53*(1), 79–85.

Brabete, A. C., & Sánchez-López, M. P. (2012). How does the gender influence people's health? Data of a sample of Romanian people living in Spain. *Procedia—Social and Behavioral Sciences, 33*, 148–152.

Craciun, B. (2013). Coping strategies, self-criticism and gender factor in relation to quality of life. *Procedia —Social and Behavioral Sciences, 78*, 466–470.

Dar, O. H., Alam, S., & Lone, Z. A. (2011). Relationship between emotional intelligence and psychological wellbeing of male police personnel. *Journal of Indian Academy of Applied Psychology, 37*(1), 47–52.

Deaux, K., & Taynor, J. (1973). Evaluation of male and female ability: Bias works two ways. *Psychological Reports, 32*(1), 261–262.

Elmer, L., MacDonald, D., & Friedman, H. (2003). Transpersonal psychology, physical health, and mental health: Theory, research and practice. *Humanistic Psychologist, 31*, 159–181.

Emmons, R. A. (2000). Is spirituality an intelligence? *The International Journal for the Psychology of Religion, 10*, 27–34.

Faribors, B., Fatemeh, A., & Hamidreza, H. (2010). The relationship between nurses' spiritual intelligence and happiness in Iran. *Procedia Social and Behavioral Sciences, 5*, 1556–1561.

Gioiella, M. E., Berkman, B., & Robinson, M. (1998). Spirituality and quality of life in gynecologic oncology patients. *Cancer Practice, 6*(6), 333–338.

Gupta, G., & Kumar, S. (2010). Mental health in relation to emotional intelligence and self-efficacy among college students. *Journal of the Indian Academy of Applied Psychology, 36*(1), 61–67.

Joshi, R., & Garg, J. M. (2013). Mental health in reference to length of service among male and female academicians. *International Journal of Research in Commerce & Management, 4*(11), 38–40.

Katyal, S., & Awasthi, E. (2005). Gender differences in emotional intelligence among adolescents of Chandigarh. *Journal of Human Ecology, 17*(2), 153–155.

Kaur, H., Singh, V., & Singh, P. (2012). Emotional intelligence: Significance of psychology and spirituality. *Pakistan Journal of Social and Clinical Psychology, 10*(1), 32–36.

Kaur, M., & Kaur, D. (2014). The power of organizational spirituality: Its effect on job satisfaction, quality of work life and occupational stress. *International Journal of Research in Organizational Behavior and Human Resource Management, 2*(2), 356–369.

Khan, I., & Singh, N. (2013). A study on gender differences on gratitude, spirituality and forgiveness among school teachers. *International Journal of Applied Sciences & Engineering, 1*(1), 9–14.

Khan, K. S. A., Vijayshri, & Farooqi, F. S. (2014). A study of religiosity in relation to spirituality and anxiety. *International Journal of Advancements in Research & Technology, 3*(4), 269–284.

Kirmani, M. N., & Suman, L. N. (2010). Gender differences in alcohol-related attitudes and expectancies among college students. *Journal of the Indian Academy of Applied Psychology, 36*(1), 19–24.

Koenig, H. G. (2004). Spirituality, wellness, and quality of life. *Sexuality, Reproduction and Menopause, 2*(2), 76–82.

Kumar, M. (2014). Study of life satisfaction among primary, middle and secondary schools teachers of district Kathua. *International Journal of Research, 1*(5), 492–498.

Kumar, S., & Bhukar, J. P. (2013). Stress level and coping strategies of college students. *Journal of Physical Education and Sports Management, 4*(1), 5–11.

Kushner, M. G., & Sher, K. J. (1993). Comorbidity of alcohol and anxiety disorders among college students: Effects of gender and family history of alcoholism. *Addictive Behaviors, 18*(5), 543–552.

Lawler, K. A., & Younger, J. W. (2002). Theobiology: An analysis of spirituality, cardiovascular responses, stress, mood, and physical health. *Journal of Religion and Health, 41*(4), 347–362.

Loewenthal, K. M., MacLeod, A. K., & Cinnirella, M. (2002). Are women more religious than men? Gender differences in religious activity among different religious groups in the UK. *Personality and Individual Differences, 32*(1), 133–139.

MacDonald, D., & Friedman, H. (2002). Assessment of humanistic, transpersonal and spiritual constructs: State of the science. *Journal of Humanistic Psychology, 42*(4), 102–125.

Megahed, M. (2014). Health-related quality of life among students at King Khalid University-Mohail Assermore. *International Journal of Nursing Science, 4*(2), 22–25.

Mercier, C., Peladeau, N., & Tempier, R. (1998). Age, gender and quality of life. *Community Mental Health Journal, 34*(5), 487–500.

Nagel, E., & Sgoutas-Emch, S. (2007). The relationship between spirituality, health beliefs, and health behaviors in college students. *Journal of Religion and Health, 46*(1), 141–154.

Naghavi, F., & Redzuan, M. (2011). The relationship between gender and emotional intelligence. *World Applied Sciences Journal, 15*(4), 555–561.

Nisa, M. (2013). Study of personality factors and family problems as determinant of mental health amongst college students. *International Journal of Advancements in Research & Technology, 2*(11), 22–32.

Pant, N., & Srivastava, S. K. (2014). Effect of spiritual intelligence on mental health and quality of life among college students. *ZENITH International Journal of Multidisciplinary Research, 4*(8), 208–215.

Pant, N., & Srivastava, S. K. (2015). Spiritual intelligence, gender and educational background as related to the quality of life of college students. *Indian Journal of Positive Psychology, 6*(3), 226–232.

Pant, N., & Srivastava, S. K. (2019). The impact of spiritual intelligence, gender and educational background on mental health among college students. *Journal of Religion and Health, 58*, 87–108.

Pardini, D. A., Plante, T. G., Sherman, A., & Stump, J. E. (2000). religious faith and spirituality in substance abuse recovery: Determining the mental health benefits. *Journal of Substance Abuse Treatment, 19*(4), 347–354.

Petrides, K. V., & Furnham, A. (2000). Gender differences in measured and self-estimated trait emotional intelligence. *Sex Roles, 42*(5–6), 449–461.

Rao, G. T. V. D., & Swathi, G. (2013). Mental health status of degree college lecturers based on gender and teaching experience in Rayalaseema Zone, Andhra Pradesh, India. *Indian Journal of Applied Research, 3*(6), 286–287.

Rippentrop, A. E., Altmaier, E. M., Chen, J. J., Found, E. M., & Kiffala, V. J. (2005). The relationship between religion/spirituality and physical health, mental health, and pain in a chronic pain population. *Journal of the International Association for the Study of Pain, 116*(3), 311–321.

Roothman, B., Kirsten, D., & Wissing, M. (2003). Gender differences in aspects of psychological well-being. *South African Journal of Psychology, 33*(4), 212–218.

Sanchez, D., & Carter, R. T. (2005). Exploring the relationship between racial identity and religious orientation among African American college students. *Journal of College Student Development, 46*(3), 280–295.

Sawatzky, R., Ratner, P. A., & Chiu, L. (2005). A meta-analysis of the relationship between spirituality and quality of life. *Social Indicators Research, 72*(2), 153–188.

Saxena, S., & Jain, R. K. (2013). Social intelligence of undergraduate students in relation to their gender and subject stream. *Journal of Research & Method in Education, 1*(1), 1–4.

Schnurr, P. P., & Lunney, C. A. (2008). Exploration of gender differences in how quality of life relates to post-traumatic stress disorder in male and female veterans. *Journal of Rehabilitation Research & Development, 45*(3), 383–394.

Sharma, V. (2014). Effect of gender and stream on depression among adolescents. *International Journal of Education and Psychological Research, 3*(2), 46–49.

Shirazi, M., & Khan, M. A. (2013). Life satisfaction among professional and non-professional students in India. *International Journal of Applied Psychology, 3*(4), 109–113.

Singh, M. P., & Sinha, J. (2013). Impact of spiritual intelligence on quality of life. *International Journal of Scientific and Research Publications, 3*(5), 1–5.

Singh, A., Kaur, P., & Singh, T. (2010). Spiritual intelligence, altruism, school environment and academic achievement as predictor of mental health of adolescents. *Journal of Exercise Science and Physiotherapy, 6*(1), 34–38.

Storrie, K., Ahern, K., & Tuckett, A. (2010). A systematic review: Students with mental health problems—A growing problem. *International Journal of Nursing Practice, 16*(1), 1–16.

Trott, D. (1996). *Spiritual well-being of workers: An exploratory study of spirituality in the workplace.* Dissertation Abstracts International, University of Texas, Austin, TX.

Walker, K. L., & Dixon, V. (2002). Spirituality and academic performance among African American college students. *Journal of Black Psychology, 28*(2), 107–121.

Wnuk, M., & Marcinkowski, J. T. (2014). Do existential variables mediate between religious-spiritual facets of functionality and psychological wellbeing? *Journal of Religion and Health, 53*(1), 56–67.

Zuckerman, D. M. (1989). Stress, self-esteem, and mental health: How does gender make a difference? *Sex Roles, 20*(78), 429–444.

Zullig, K. J., Ward, R. M., & Horn, T. (2006). The association between perceived spirituality, religiosity, and life satisfaction: The mediating role of self-rated health. *Social Indicators Research, 79*(2), 255274.

Chapter 4
The Role of Spirituality in Predicting Mental Health and Quality of Life Among Early Adults

This chapter includes the author's own studies and research which explore and investigate the role of spirituality in predicting mental health and quality of life among early adults. Where past research and studies were conducted with mixed constructs and concepts, which did not effectively contrast spirituality and religiosity, this study utilizes the latest concept of spiritual intelligence, is conducted in an Indian setting and plays a key role in understanding the role of spirituality in enhancing mental health and quality of life among early adults. This chapter presents the author's research, designed to examine the role of spirituality in predicting mental health and quality of life among early adults. The chapter first outlines the objectives and hypotheses of the study, then describes the methodology, followed by presentation of the results and discussion, and finally, a summary of the findings and conclusion.

4.1 Objectives and Hypotheses of the Study

These objectives were determined based on the findings of past studies and on the focus of the present study. The following hypotheses were formulated on the basis of these objectives.

4.1.1 Objectives

1. To identify the effect of spirituality on mental health among early adults.
2. To identify the effect of spirituality on quality of life (QoL) among early adults.

N. Pant, *Spirituality, Mental Health and Quality of Life*,
https://doi.org/10.1007/978-981-99-2703-6_4

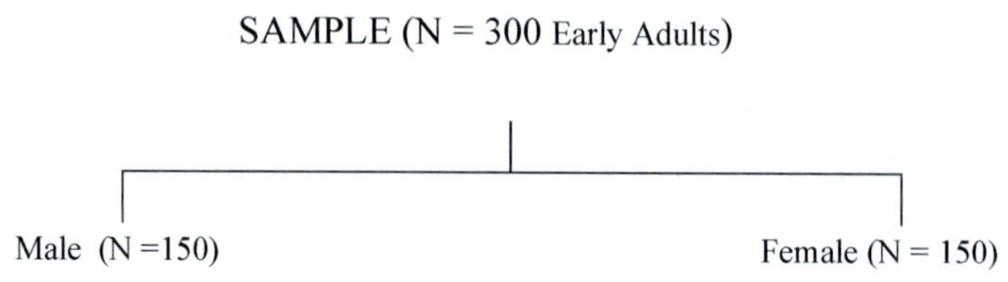

Fig. 4.1 Showing the distribution of early adults on the basis of gender

4.1.2 Hypotheses

1. There would be a significant effect of spiritual intelligence on mental health among early adults.
2. There would be a significant effect of spiritual intelligence on QoL among early adults.

4.2 Methodology

4.2.1 Selection of Sample

The correlational design is the basis of the current research. A purposive sample of 300 early adults (150 male and 150 female) was selected as a sample for the study (see Fig. 4.1). The data were collected from four different government degree colleges and campuses in the Haridwar district of Uttarakhand, India. The age range of the early adults chosen for the sample was from 20 to 30 years.

Tools/scales were administered to the sample of early adults during college hours by the researcher. They were assured of the complete confidentiality of their responses and the importance of accurate responses was emphasized.

4.2.2 Use of Psychological Tools/Scales

The following tools/scales were used for the collection of data:

Personal **B**io-data Sheet:

This is on the cover of the entire booklet (questionnaire), where the individual(participant) enters his or her personal information. Instructions, and spaces for the participant's name, gender, age and educational information are all included on this cover.

The Integrated Spiritual Intelligence Scale (ISIS): This 83-item self-report questionnaire, developed by Amram and Dryer (2008), offers scores for five broad categories and 22 specific capabilities (see Table 4.1), in addition to a single, overall assessment of spiritual intelligence (SI). The ISIS demonstrates acceptable test/retest reliability: Pearson $r = 0.77, p < 0.01$. The convergent and discriminant validity of this scale is very good in relation with various other related scales and groups. A high score on this measure denotes high spiritual intelligence. This scale explains the creation and initial validation of the Integrated Spiritual Intelligence Scale, an ecumenical measure of spiritual intelligence (SI), defined as the ability to apply, manifest and embody spiritual resources, values and qualities to enhance daily functioning and wellbeing. It contains 22 subscales assessing separate SI capabilities related to Beauty, Discernment, Egolessness, Equanimity, Freedom, Gratitude, Higher-self, Holism, Immanence, Inner-wholeness, Intuition, Joy, Mindfulness, Openness, Practice, Presence, Purpose, Relatedness, Sacredness, Service, Synthesis and Trust. As mentioned earlier, these 22 subscales are grouped into five domains: Consciousness, Grace, Meaning, Transcendence and Truth. The ISIS correlated with existing spirituality measures and predicted life satisfaction. Even after adjusting for other confounding factors, there were substantial differences in ISIS ratings between the various groups, with business leaders and spiritual teachers who were recognized for embodying spirituality in daily life scoring higher than MBA students.

The scale defines spiritual intelligence as a set of abilities that people can use to apply, embody and manifest spiritual resources, ideals and traits in ways that improve daily life and welfare. These skills are present in people to varying degrees, and practice or training may aid in the development of some or all of these skills. Amram and Dryer (2008) group these abilities into five broad domains of spiritual intelligence:

1. *Consciousness.* In order to improve daily functioning and wellbeing, this domain reflects the capacity to raise or shift consciousness, access intuition, and synthesize many points of view. Three capabilities were identified within the consciousness domain: Intuition, Mindfulness and Synthesis.
2. *Grace.* In order to improve functioning and wellbeing, this domain draws on the inspiration, beauty and joy that are available in every moment and represent inner-directedness (combining discernment and freedom). Six capabilities of grace were identified: Beauty, Discernment, Freedom, Gratitude, Immanence and Joy.
3. *Meaning.* This domain shows the capacity to create interpretations that improve functioning and welfare even in the face of pain and suffering. Furthermore this demonstrates the experience of meaning, values, and the link activities. Purpose and Service are the two capabilities of meaning.
4. *Transcendence.* This domain demonstrates the capacity to transcend the egoic self and align with the sacred in ways that improve functioning and wellbeing. The five capabilities of transcendence are Higher-self, Holism, Practice, Relatedness and Sacredness.
5. *Truth.* This domain displays open receptivity, presence, humility, and trust in ways that improve daily functioning and wellbeing. It exhibits the capacity to be present to, love and peacefully surrender to truth. Egolessness, Equanimity,

Table 4.1 List of five domains with their 22 capabilities (subscales) of ISIS

Domain	Capability no	Capability/Subscale	No. of items
1. Consciousness	1	Intuition	4
	2	Mindfulness	5
	3	Synthesis	3
2. Grace	4	Beauty	3
	5	Discernment	4
	6	Freedom	3
	7	Gratitude	2
	8	Immanence	4
	9	Joy	3
3. Meaning	10	Purpose	5
	11	Service	3
4. Transcendence	12	Higher-Self	5
	13	Holism	4
	14	Practice	6
	15	Relatedness	3
	16	Sacredness	4
5. Truth	17	Egolessness	3
	18	Equanimity	3
	19	Inner-Wholeness	4
	20	Openness	4
	21	Presence	3
	22	Trust	4

Items no. 2, 7, 9, 11, 13, 18, 22, 23, 26, 31, 33, 44, 53, 55, 60, 63, 74, 75, 76, 78, 79 and 81 (total 22) are reverse items in the scale

Inner-wholeness, Openness, Presence, and Trust are the six capabilities that make up truth.

Despite the positive psychometric qualities mentioned above for the ISIS, this scale has a number of limitations. The scale was the first of its sort, and to support the published findings, no replication studies demonstrating generalizability with diverse populations have been carried out. As noted by the developers of the scale, the factor structure and different psychometric features, in particular, should only be viewed as preliminary. Further, they suggest that future research is necessary to show the predictive validity of the ISIS, beyond subjective wellbeing, and its discriminant validity in comparison with other well-established constructs like emotional intelligence and personality. Additionally, spiritual intelligence is a multidimensional construct with many different aspects, themes and sub-themes. Therefore, it is unclear whether the existing 22 capability subscales and five domain scales of ISIS accurately represent all facets of spiritual intelligence.

Mithila Mental Health Status Inventory (MMHSI): The 50 items on this scale, which has five subscales, are written both positively and negatively. The Hindi adaptation of MMHSI was developed by Kumar and Thakur (1986). The inventory's split-half and test/retest reliability are, respectively, 0.90 and 0.87. The test was developed on both normal students and psychiatric patients to determine concurrent validity. On all five subscales, the difference was statistically significant and there was a strong association between these results and the Eysenck Personality Questionnaire (EPQ). Poor mental health is indicated by a high score on this scale. Following is a brief summary of the five subscales:

1. *The egocentrism scale* measures how much a person is focused on his or her own needs, feelings, views and ideas. High scorers on this scale would have trouble empathizing with or identifying with other people. A high score on this scale also suggests a tendency to withdraw, which makes it harder maintain interpersonal relationships.
2. *The alienation scale* was designed to show how much the respondent resembled hospitalized psychiatric patients. High scorers on this measure would exhibit suspicious behaviour, excessive sensitivity, unusual sensations and sensory distortions.
3. *The expression scale* measures how socially interactive a group of individuals are. High ratings on this scale imply a lack of social disclosure, inconsistent relationships in social settings and a sense of insecurity.
4. *The emotional instability measure* shows how unhappy, nervous, emotionally brittle, afraid, anxious or depressed the person is. A high rating on this scale suggests that the person has significant personality issues and would require psychological and psychiatric support. Such individuals will undoubtedly experience adjustment issues.
5. *The social non-conformity measure* indicates whether the person aligns with or against the current social system. People who score highly on this measure are likely to be narcissistic. These individuals are reluctant to participate effectively in common social situations.

World Health Organization Quality of Life Scale (WHOQOL-BREF):

The WHOQOL-BREF field trial version was created to offer a short form, quality of life assessment because the WHOQOL-100 was too long for practical application. The 26 items of the WHOQOL-BREF measure these four broad domains: physical health, psychological health, social relationships and environment. One item from each of the 24 facets included in the WHOQOL-100 has been included in this scale to offer a broad and thorough assessment. In addition, two items from the facets of general health and overall quality of life have been added. A high rating on this scale denotes a high quality of life.

4.2.3 Procedure

Every participant chosen as part of the sample received a personal copy of the questionnaire booklet. All participants were made aware that the booklet was to be completed anonymously and their answers would be treated confidentially. They were asked to complete the booklet in accordance with the instructions printed therein. Each participant turned in a completed booklet, which was collected. They finished the booklet in between 30 and 60 min. Data collected was examined. The questionnaires with blank spaces were not included in the analyses.

4.2.4 Statistical Techniques Used

In light of the study's objectives and hypotheses, the collected data on the various scales were analysed. Mean and SD were used for descriptive analyses, Pearson Correlation was adopted for analysing correlation, and regression analysis methods were employed for analysing effects. Microsoft Excel and SPSS, two more pieces of software, were used to complete all of the statistical analyses.

4.3 Results and Discussion

This study is designed to observe the role of spirituality in predicting mental health and quality of life among early adults. Results have been arranged in accordance with the stated objectives and hypotheses of the study. First, this section explores the mean values and standard deviation of the three constructs: spiritual intelligence (SI), mental health (MH) and quality of life (QOL). Then, the outcomes are explained in light of the hypotheses.

As mentioned in the tools and scales section, higher scores on the ISIS (Spiritual Intelligence Scale) indicate high spiritual intelligence, while high scores on the MMHSI (Mental Health Scale) indicate poor mental health. High scores on the WHOQOL-BREF (Quality of Life Scale) indicate good quality of life. Table 4.2 shows the mean values and SDs of 300 early adults' scores on these three scales. The scores were 326.01 mean value and 34.89 SD on the ISIS, 129.64 mean value and 13.39 SD on the MMHSI, and 90.22 mean value and 12.04 SD on the WHOQOL-BREF scale (Pant & Srivastava, 2015, 2019). This indicates good similarity with the scales' norms and good variance on the normal probability curve. This represents the graphical normality of the data.

Hypothesis 1 There would be a significant effect of spiritual intelligence on mental health among early adults.

In Hypothesis 1 it was posited that a significant effect of spiritual intelligence on mental health among early adults would be observed. The results of the study mean

Table 4.2 Showing the mean values and standard deviation for the SI, MH and QOL

Constructs	*N*	Minimum	Maximum	Mean	Standard deviation (SD)
SI (Spiritual Intelligence)	300	213.00	435.00	326.01	34.89
MH (Mental Health)	300	99.00	160.00	129.64	13.39
QOL (Quality of Life)	300	54.00	121.00	90.22	12.04

Table 4.3 Showing the correlation and regression between spiritual intelligence and mental health of early adults

	N	SI		MH		Correlation coefficient (*r*)	*R* Square
		Mean	SD	Mean	SD		
Total	300	326.01	34.89	129.64	13.39	**0.553***	**0.306****
Male	150	323.95	40.43	129.37	14.19	0.576*	0.332**
Female	150	328.07	28.27	129.91	12.59	0.531*	0.282**

*p-value < 0.01 (2-tailed), **F is significant at 0.01 level

this hypothesis is accepted and suggest that spiritual intelligence significantly affects mental health among early adults. There is a highly significant correlation (0.553) between the SI and MH of early adults. This means that as the degree of spiritual intelligence increases, the level of poor mental health decreases. Regression analysis predicts 30.6% chances (0.306) of spiritual intelligence causing variance in mental health among the sample of early adults, which is significant at 0.01 level. So, there is no doubt the hypothesis is accepted. Table 4.3 shows the scores of 300 early adults (150 male and 150 female) on both SI and MH scales. Where the mean value and SD of 300 early adults on SI are respectively 326.01 and 34.89, the mean value and SD on MH are respectively 129.64 and 13.39. Further, separately, Table 3.3 shows a high significant correlation (0.576) and *R* Square (0.332) between SI and MH of 150 male early adults and a high significant correlation (0.531) and *R* Square (0.282) between SI and MH of 150 female early adults.

These results are supported by other research studies. A study by Edmondson et al. (2005) of 52 female participants from various cultural and socioeconomic backgrounds, looked into the effects of spirituality and religiosity on self-reported physical health. According to their findings, existential wellbeing is linked to lower mean heart rates and less heartrate reactivity, as well as fewer physical health complaints. Reduced systolic blood pressure reactivity in response to the structured interview is linked to religious wellbeing. These results imply that spirituality may benefit health, even in a group of very young individuals. Nagel and Sgoutas-Emch (2007) used measures of both spirituality and religion in a study of college students in the United States to investigate if the same pattern of relationships observed previously is visible in a sample of healthy college students. They also looked at health-related behaviours and beliefs. Their findings indicate that those who scored higher on spirituality are more active and have different health beliefs than people who scored lower on spirituality. Alihosseini et al. (2014), in their study of the relationship between spiritual intelligence and its component units and happiness in young people, discovered that there is a positive and significant relation between spiritual intelligence and its component units (like inner peace, spiritual experiences, forgiveness and self-awareness) and happiness. Further study of the effect of spiritual intelligence on college students' mental health and quality of life was conducted by Pant and Srivastava (2014). The study's conclusions showed a significant association between spiritual intelligence and mental health, a significant relationship between spiritual intelligence and quality of life, and a significant relationship between mental health and quality of life among college students. Furthermore, college students' mental health was examined by Pant and Srivastava (2019) in relation to their spiritual intelligence, gender and educational background. It discovered that there is a considerable link between spiritual intelligence and mental health among students who study the arts, with the relationship also being separate for male and female students. Students studying science have a strong association between spiritual intelligence and mental health, and there is also a separate significant relationship among male and female science students (Fig. 4.2).

Hypothesis 2 There would be a significant effect of spiritual intelligence on QoL among early adults.

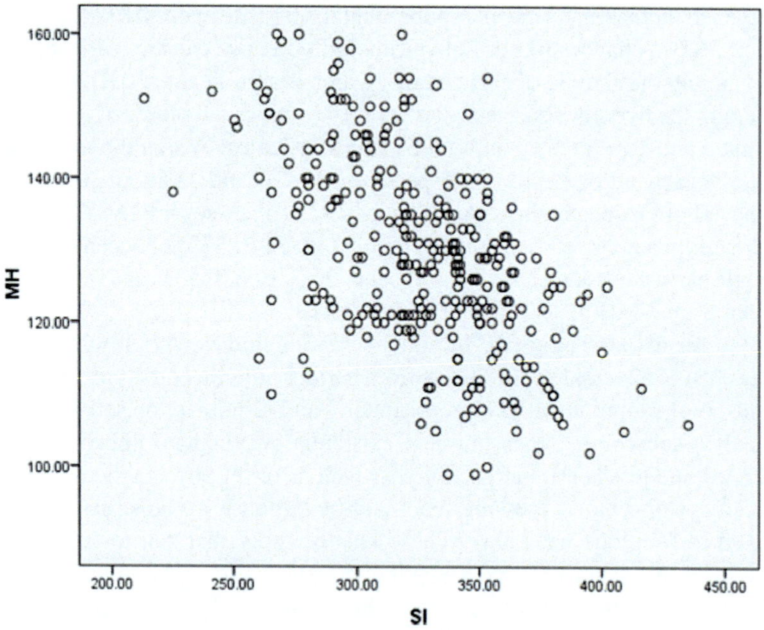

Fig. 4.2 Showing the relationship between spiritual intelligence and mental health of early adults ($N = 300$) (X axis: SI (Spiritual Intelligence Scores), Y axis: MH [Mental Health Scores])

In Hypothesis 2 it was posited that a significant effect of spiritual intelligence on QOL among early adults would be observed. As previously, the results of the study mean that this hypothesis is accepted and suggest that spiritual intelligence and QOL relate significantly among early adults. There is a high significant correlation (0.498) between the SI and QOL of early adults. This means that as the degree of spiritual intelligence increases, the level of QOL increases. Regression analysis predicts 24.8% chances (0.248) of spiritual intelligence causing variance in quality of life among the sample of early adults, which is significant at 0.01 level. So, there is no doubt this hypothesis is also accepted. Table 4.4 shows the scores of 300 early adults (150 male and 150 female) on both SI and QoL scales of. Where the mean value and SD of 300 early adults on SI are respectively 326.01 and 34.89, the mean value and SD on QOL are respectively 90.22 and 12.04. Further, separately, Table 3.4 shows the high significant correlation (0.532) and R Square (0.283) between the SI and QOL of 150 male early adults, and high significant correlation (0.472) and R Square (0.223) between the SI and QOL of 150 female early adults. Many previous studies and research support these results. The same scale of QOL was used in Teichmann et al.'s (2006) study on spiritual needs and quality of life in Estonia, and their findings indicate that spirituality plays a significant role in a person's view of their quality of life in a changing socioeconomic environment. Ahmadi et al. (2012) looked into the relationship between life quality and spiritual intelligence and taking some responsibility. According to the research findings, transcendental awareness, one of the subscales of spiritual intelligence, accounts for a greater proportion of the life quality of the students when it comes to explaining that quality. Consequently, as transcendental awareness increases, so does the influence it has on life quality. Singh and Sinha (2013) conducted research to determine the effect of spiritual intelligence on the quality of life of government organization executives. They discovered that, in the majority of cases where SQ (spiritual intelligence) was high, QOL was greater. Further research into the effect of spiritual intelligence on college students' mental health and quality of life was conducted by Pant and Srivastava (2014). The study's conclusions showed a significant association between spiritual intelligence and mental health, a significant relationship between spiritual intelligence and quality of life, and a significant relationship between mental health and quality of life among college students. Further research on spiritual intelligence, gender, and educational background as they relate to college students' quality of life was conducted by Pant and Srivastava (2015). This study's conclusions showed that spiritual intelligence and quality of life are substantially correlated among arts students, with significant correlations for both male and female arts students. In science students, there is a considerable association between spiritual intelligence and quality of life; this relationship is present for both male and female science students (Fig. 4.3).

Table 4.4 Showing the correlation and regression between spiritual intelligence and QOL of early adults

	N	SI		QoL		Correlation coefficient (*r*)	*R* Square
		Mean	SD	Mean	SD		
TOTAL	300	326.01	34.89	90.22	12.04	**0.498***	**0.248****
Male	150	323.95	40.43	90.50	12.14	0.532*	0.283**
Female	150	328.07	28.27	89.93	11.97	0.472*	0.223**

*p-value < 0.01 (2-tailed), **F is significant at 0.01 level

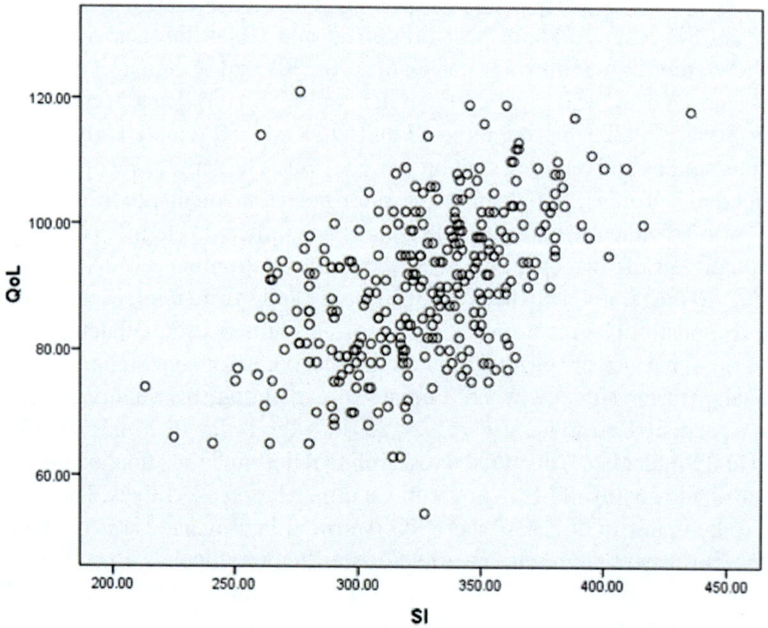

Fig. 4.3 Showing the relationship between spiritual intelligence and QOL of early adults (N = 300) (X axis: SI (Spiritual Intelligence Scores), Y axis: QoL [Quality of Life Scores])

4.4 Summary and Conclusion

The main purposes of the study, as the chapter title indicates, were to observe the role of spirituality in predicting mental health and quality of life among early adults. After reviewing works done both in India and worldwide, two research questions were raised in the study: (1) Is there any significant effect of spiritual intelligence on mental health among early adults? (2) Is there any significant effect of spiritual intelligence on quality of life among early adults? Two hypotheses were developed to investigate these objectives. The sample of early adults were chosen from several colleges in Haridwar, India, for the data collection. Three scales were used to assess spiritual intelligence, mental health and quality of life, including the Integrated Spiritual

Intelligence Scale (ISIS), the Mithila Mental Health Status Inventory (MMHSI), and the WHOQOL-BREF. All of the scores were listed following the data collection. The Pearson correlation method was used to analyse relationships, while simple regression methods are used to analyse effects. The statistical analysis software SPSS was used for all calculations. Findings of the regression revealed that spiritual intelligence is a significant predictor of mental health and quality of life among early adults, which determines a significant effect of spiritual intelligence on mental health and quality of life among early adults. Correlational analyses revealed that there is a significant positive relationship between spiritual intelligence and mental health and a significant positive relationship between spiritual intelligence and QOL among early adults. Furthermore, male and female early adults separately showed significant positive relationships and effects between spiritual intelligence and mental health and significant positive relationship and effects between spiritual intelligence and QOL. In both, the results of relationships and effects were stronger in males than females.

4.4.1 Limitations of the Study

The study also showed the following limitations:

1. The sample was only representative of the city of Haridwar; it would be appropriate if it included residents of other states and districts across the nation.
2. The Mithila Mental Health Status Inventory (MMHSI), a measure of mental health, is not the best currently available option, and not very suitable for the current scenario.
3. Only early adults in the general population were included in the study's sample; it would be more appropriate to include spiritual practitioners as well.
4. The study was limited to constructs as a whole; it would be more valuable if the study focused on separate dimensions of the constructs.

4.4.2 Recommendations for Future Research

Researchers and mental health professionals can learn a lot from the conclusions of this study regarding the importance of spirituality (or spiritual intelligence) for improving mental health and quality of life. Future researchers are urged to put the following recommendations into practice when repeating these kinds of studies:

1. To achieve better results, it would be imperative to employ a contemporary, standardized mental health scale.
2. It would be more beneficial for the researcher to choose a sample from the many cities and states around the nation to include both rural and urban populations.
3. If the sample for a research study on spirituality was also drawn from the population of spiritual practitioners, the study would be stronger.

4. Only the early adult age group is represented in the sample of the current study, which was drawn from colleges and campuses. In order to conduct a cross-sectional study, it is advisable that the future researcher choose a sample from the middle and late adult groups.
5. Future studies are advised to make some firm predictions in order to support the relevance of spirituality in the context of mental health. For this, researchers are advised to select more well-developed scales and all dimensions of spirituality and spiritual intelligence in the study.
6. The research would be more useful if it was conducted in an experimental context.

4.4.3 Conclusion

Finally, the study reaches the conclusion that spiritual intelligence is a significant predictor of mental health and quality of life among early adults, which determines a significant effect of spiritual intelligence on mental health and quality of life among early adults. There is a significant positive relationship between spiritual intelligence and mental health and a significant positive relationship between spiritual intelligence and QOL among early adults. Furthermore, male and female early adults separately have shown significant positive relationships and effects between spiritual intelligence and mental health and significant positive relationship and effects between spiritual intelligence and QOL. In all the results, relationships and effects were stronger in males than females. So, on the basis of prior research and the results of the present study, finally it may be concluded that spirituality in the form of spiritual intelligence might be impactful in improving mental health and quality of life.

Disclosure of Conflicts of Interest/Funding Information
There is no conflict of interest regarding the study. All procedures performed in studies involving human participants were in accordance with the ethical standards and adherence to the legal requirements. This research does not contain any studies with animals conducted by the author. The author has no funding to report.

References

Ahmadi, A., Ahghar, G., & Abedi, M. R. (2012). The relationship between spiritual intelligence and taking responsibility with life quality. *European Online Journal of Natural and Social Sciences, 2*(3), 391–400.

Alihosseini, F., Rangan, U., Alihosseini, A., & Hajmohammadi, F. (2014). A study of the relationship between spiritual intelligence and its components with happiness in youths. *The International Journal of Humanities & Social Studies, 2*(6), 56–60.

Amram, Y., & Dryer, D. C. (2008, August 14–17). *The integrated spiritual intelligence scale (ISIS): Development and preliminary validation.* Paper presented at the 116th Annual Conference of the American Psychological Association, Boston, MA.

Edmondson, K. A., Lawler, K. A., Jobe, R. L., Younger, J. W., Piferi, R. L., & Jones, W. H. (2005). Spirituality predicts health and cardiovascular responses to stress in young adult women. *Journal of Religion and Health, 44*(2), 161–171.

Kumar, A., & Thakur, G. P. (1986). *Mithila mental health status inventory (MMHSI).* Ganga Saran and Grand Sons.

Nagel, E., & Sgoutas-Emch, S. (2007). The relationship between spirituality, health beliefs, and health behaviors in college students. *Journal of Religion and Health, 46*(1), 141–154.

Pant, N., & Srivastava, S. K. (2014). Effect of spiritual intelligence on mental health and quality of life among college students. *ZENITH International Journal of Multidisciplinary Research, 4*(8), 208–215.

Pant, N., & Srivastava, S. K. (2015). Spiritual intelligence, gender and educational background as related to the quality of life of college students. *Indian Journal of Positive Psychology, 6*(3), 226–232.

Pant, N., & Srivastava, S. K. (2019). The impact of spiritual intelligence, gender and educational background on mental health among college students. *Journal of Religion and Health, 58*, 87–108.

Singh, M. P., & Sinha, J. (2013). Impact of spiritual intelligence on quality of life. *International Journal of Scientific and Research Publications, 3*(5), 1–5.

Teichmann, M., Murdvee, M., & Saks, K. (2006). Spiritual needs and quality of life in Estonia. *Social Indicators Research, 76*(1), 147–163.

Chapter 5
Indian Psychology of Mind and Mental Health

As per Indian psychology (philosophy), the ultimate goal of life is to achieve ultimate truth ('paramatma'). To attain this goal, a healthy body and a healthy mind are needed. An Indian scholar, Maharshi Charaka in his famous work *Charaka Samhita* described the importance of health ('aarogya'):

> धर्मार्थकामोक्षाणांमारोग्यम मूलमुत्तमम्
> Dharmarthkaamokshaanaamarogyam moolmuttamam,
> रोगास्तस्यापहर्तारः श्रेयसो जीवितस्य च
> Rogastsyaphartarah shreyaso jeevitasya cha.
> प्रादुर्भूतो मनुष्याणामन्तरायो महानयम
> Pradurbhooto manusyanaamntaraayoo mahaanayam,
> कः स्याक्तेशां भामोपाय इत्युक्त्वा ध्यानमास्थिताः
> Kah syakteshaam bhamopay ityuktwa dhyanmasthitaa.
>
> Essence: The foremost quest of mankind is health. Fulfilment of all goals either worldly or spiritual is dependent on health.
>
> *Charaka Samhita*/Sutra Sthan – 15, 16

5.1 Concepts of Health and Mental Health in Indian Psychology

In Ayurvedic science, health and ill health are the results of the kind of food an individual consumes. Further, even if a good quality of food is ingested it cannot amount to wellbeing until it is properly digested and assimilated. Thus, good health depends on both the quality and quantity of food ingested, as well as the body's capability to assimilate it. This capability or power of assimilation is called 'agni' in Ayurvedic medicine. 'Agni' is described as 'jathragni' at the level of digestion, and 'dhatwagni' and 'bhutagni' at the level of assimilation. Indian psychology defines health ('swasthya') as an Ayurvedic approach indicating health as a balance in 'tridoshas',

N. Pant, *Spirituality, Mental Health and Quality of Life*,
https://doi.org/10.1007/978-981-99-2703-6_5

13 'agnis' (flames or metabolic fires), 7 'dhatus' (tissues), and in the eliminating processes of waste products, and finally it is defined as the happiness of 'atma' (the soul or consciousness), the five senses and the mind –

> समदोषः समाग्निश्च समधातुमलक्रियः।
> Samdosah samagnisch samdhatumalkriyah,
> प्रसन्नात्मेन्द्रियमनाः स्वस्थ इत्यभिधीयते।।
> Prasannatmendriyamana swasth ityabhidheeyate.
>
> Balance in 'vata', 'pitta' and 'kapha' ('doshas'), flames or metabolic fires ('agni'), tissues ('dhatu'), eliminating processes of waste products ('malkriya') and happiness of soul or consciousness ('aatama') and senses is called health ('swasthya')
>
> *Shushruta Samhita*, 15/41.

Ayurveda accepts health as a *balance* of biological and psychological aspects. There are three major mental diseases described in the famous text the *Raamcharitmanas*; 'kaam' (false desire), 'krodh' (anger) and 'lobh' (greed), which are caused by an imbalance in the 'tridoshas': 'vata', 'pitta', and 'kapha'. In this way, this definition of health covers all aspects. There are three 'gunas' (natures) which also need to be in equilibrium to make an individual healthy: 'sattva' (the element of illumination), 'rajas' (activity, dynamism), and 'tamas' (passivity, darkness). Such a balanced state of functioning is repeatedly considered in the *Bhagvad Gita* to be the chief characteristic of the psychological wellbeing of a person (Palsane et al., 1986; Sinha, 1990).

Ayurveda defines mental health as a state of mental, intellectual and spiritual wellbeing. According to the *Bhagvad Gita*, the three mental diseases discussed earlier are the result of 'rajas guna' (Gita 3/37). Besides this, we have an unlimited source of knowledge on spirituality and mental/physical health from an Indian perspective in *Charaka Samhita*, *Sushruta Samhita* and other books on Ayurveda as well as *Sad-darshanas* and many other books. According to *Charaka Samhita* (Sutra Sthan) 'vata', 'pitta' and 'kapha' are three physical disorders and 'rajas' and 'tamas' are two mental disorders. According to this text, the third 'sattva guna' is not a disorder but a good nature needed for mental health.

To attain good physical and mental health the major requirements emphasized in Ayurveda are: a balanced diet plan ('haar'), enough sleep ('nidra'/'swapn'), and control over material desires ('brahmacharya').

> त्रय उपस्तंभा इति आहारः स्वप्नो ब्रह्मचर्यमिति
> Traya upastambha iti aharah swapno brahmcharyamiti.
>
> *'Aahar' (diet) is one of the factors of 'traya upastambha', others being 'nidra' and 'brmhacharya'*
>
> *Charaka Samhita* (Sutra Sthan – 11/35).

Modern psychology assumes mental health to be the absence of psychological diseases, or the presence of psychological wellbeing. And Indian psychology assumes mental illness to be the increase in the 'rajoguna' and the 'tamoguna'. According to the *Charaka Samhita* (Sutra Sthan 1/56):

'Vata', 'pitta' and 'kapha' are physical disorders and 'rajoguna' and 'tamoguna' are mental disorders'

Charaka Samhita (Sutra Sthan – 1/56).

Similarly, in the *Mahabharata* (Santiparva 16/13) mental health is defined as:

सत्वं रजस्तम इति मानसाः स्युस्त्रयो गुणाः

satvam rajastam iti maanasaah syustrayo gunaah,

तेषां गुणानां साम्यं यक्त दाहुः स्वस्थलक्षणम्

tesam gunanam saamyam yakt daahuh swasthlakshanam.

'Sattva', 'raja' and 'tama' are three mental traits. The balancing state of the three traits is the state of actual mental health

Mahabharata (Santiparva 16/13).

A major cause of all physical problems is mental illness, as is found in modern and ancient studies. Frequently occurring and observable problems of the current time are a faulty lifestyle and an aimless life. The goals of many in society have become economic success and material fun. This is supported by Bhagvan Shree Krishna in the *Bhagvad Gita*:

ध्यायतो विष्यान्पुन्सः संगस्तेषूप्जायते

Dhyayato vishyanpunsah sangasteshoopjaayate,

संगात्संजायते कामः कामात्क्रोधोभिजायते

Sangaatsanjaayate kaamah kaamaatkrodhobhijayate.

Essence: The origination of diseases is only due to lust of human being for life and the physical world. Disease originates because of faulty lifestyles and perceptions.

Bhagvad Gita, 2/62

When discussing the character of Shree Krishna, we observe it is full of psychological phenomena. When Arjun denied fighting the war against his relatives in Kurukshetra, then Bhagvan Shree Krishna blessed him with the 'gita gyan' to fight with his mind set up. This is why 'Gita' is also thought of as a therapy (CBT) among Indian psychologists (Sharma, 2014).

Indian psychology and Indian philosophy have a huge range of material on health, mental health and related aspects. Leading texts include: *Yoga*, *Upanishad*, *Gita* and *Vedanta*, among others. The *Patanjali Yogasutra* is the leading text of Mahamuni Patanjali, which also describes psychological concepts alongside their clinical use. Singh (1986) also finds Yoga to be a 'potent tool of mental health promotion'. The famous and root 'sutra' of *Patanjali Yogasutra* is where Yoga is explained as:

योगश्च चित्तवृत्ति निरोधः।

Yogashchittavrittinirodhah.

Yoga is restraining the mind-stuff ('chitta') from taking various forms ('vrttis')

Patanjali Yogasutra, 1/2.

A famous saying is: 'No health without mental health' but I will further add: 'No mental health without spiritual health.' Spiritual health comes in life when individuals live their lives in spiritual ways. Further, if seeking to find spirituality described in Indian philosophy, the core theory in studying the subject is Advaita Vedanata. The Advaita concept is based on the spiritual dimension of wholeness and Oneness.

5.2 Structure and Dynamics of Personality in Indian Psychology

As in modern psychology, Indian psychology has a large amount of study material in the field of the psychology of personality, and the psychology of the mind and mental health. Although a century has passed since the emergence of psychology as a science, even now we haven't reached agreement on the structure and dynamics of personality and mind. How can it be possible to study mental health and the mind and cure mental illness without detailed knowledge and understanding and a final judgement on the structural and dynamic parts of the mind and personality? That is why this section will try to view the concepts of mind, mental health and personality from an Indian psychological perspective. In the *Upanishads*, it is told that the 'jeeva' (self) lies in five 'koshas' (sheaths) (see Fig. 5.1):

1. **'Annamaya Kosha' (Physical Sheath)**: This includes the senses and the body; it indicates the physical appearance of the 'jeeva' (organism) and is constructed by food.
2. **'Pranmaya Kosha' (Energy Sheath)**: This is the body's inbuilt vital and driving forces; the body remains in existence because of this 'prana' power.
3. **'Manomaya Kosha' (Mind/Mental Sheath)**: This sheath indicates mind and mental 'sankalp' (will).

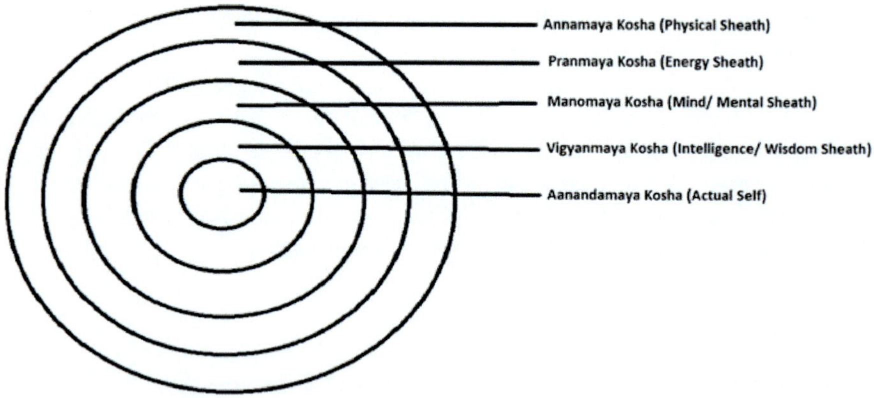

Fig. 5.1 The five koshas (Sheaths)

4. **'Vigyanmaya Kosha' (Intelligence/Wisdom Sheath)**: This sheath includes 'buddhi' (intelligence) and its functions. It has the sense of dualism.
5. **'Aanandamaya Kosha' (Actual Self/Bliss Sheath)**: This has the sense of non-dualism and limitless bliss. Beyond the false sense of self, it is the actual spiritual self.

Because the 'man' (mind) lies in between the Pranmaya and Vigyanmaya Koshas, that is why it is necessary for both 'karma' (body functions) and 'gyan' (intelligence). There are two 'karanas' (sources) in the 'jeeva' (organism): 'bahya'(outer) 'karan' and 'antah' (inside) 'karan'. The 'gyanendri' (five senses) and 'karmendri' (mouth, hands, feet, anus and genitals) are the 'bahya' (outer) 'karan'. On other hand 'man' (mind), 'ahankara' (sense of bodily self) and 'buddhi' (intelligence) are the 'antah' (inside) 'karan'. As per the *Chhandogya Upanishad,* the food we consume is converted into three forms: the waste and most dense part is converted into stool; the average part is converted into muscles and the micro part is converted into 'manas' (mind). So, the importance of good, light food for good mental health is emphasized in the *Chhandogya Upanished* and *Bhagvad Gita.* In its 15th chapter, the *Bhagvad Gita* explains the 'man' (mind) as the sixth sense. Some scholars explain this *Bhagvad Gita* theory of 'man' (mind) as being beyond the senses, so we can say that 'man' (mind) lies beyond the senses, 'buddhi' (intelligence) lies beyond the 'man' (mind), and finally, 'atma' (self) lies beyond 'buddhi' (intelligence).

5.2.1 Indian Model of Personality

In psychoanalysis Sigmund Freud (1957) illustrated the structure of personality as made up of the Conscious, Subconscious and Unconscious, and the dynamics of personality as being the Id, Ego and Superego. Likewise, Indian psychology explains the dynamics of the personality as a chariot. As per the *Kathopnishad* (1st chapter, 3rd Valli, 3–4th Shloka), the 'atma' (self) is illustrated as the lord of the chariot (passenger), 'buddhi' (intelligence) is portrayed as the 'saarathi' (charioteer), 'man' (mind) as the 'lagaam' (reins) and the 'gyanendri' (senses) as the five horses of the body chariot. The *Maitrayani Upanishad* explains the 'man' (mind) as the charioteer, the senses as the 'lagaam' (reins), and the 'karmendri' (mouth, hands, feet, anus and genitals) as the five horses of the body chariot. Figure 5.2 illustrates the chariot as the physical body, the five horses of the chariot as the five 'karmendri' (mouth, hands, feet, anus and genitals) to perform the action, the reins as the five senses to perceive the objects, the charioteer as the 'antah karan' (mind, intellect and bodily self) to exert control over the senses and 'karmendri'. The whip in the hands of charioteer is the 'vivek' (discretion) to prevent the horses going the wrong way, or, in other words the 'vivek' (discretion) prevents the senses and the 'karmendri' from going to the wrong places or taking the wrong paths; it helps 'antah karan' to make choices: yes or no, good or bad, noble or wrong. Finally, Fig. 5.2 illustrates the passenger or the lord of the chariot as the 'jeeva atma' (individualized self), which is the cause

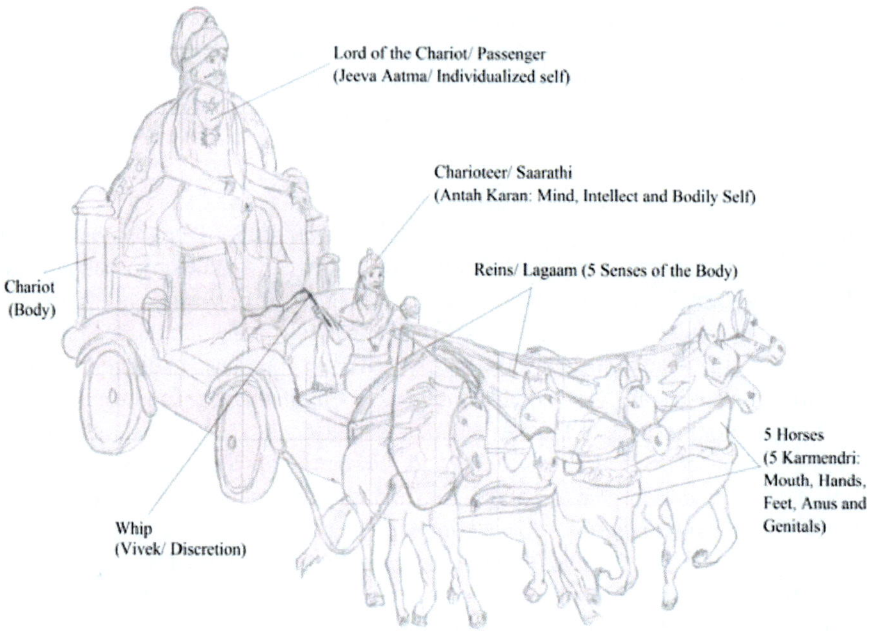

Fig. 5.2 Chariot illustrating the dynamics of personality (Indian Model of Personality)

of the body. Similar to this model of dynamics of the personality, we find other similar concepts of three 'sareeras' (bodies) in Indian psychology (i.e., in *Samkhya Darshan* and others), which describes three bodies to be 'sthool sareer' (physical body), 'sooksma sareer' (subtle body) and 'karan sareer' (causal body).

5.3 Managing Self: Indian Perspective

5.3.1 Self in Modern Science

In psychology the self is an archetype that works with the ego to manage other archetypes and balance the personality (Ciccarelli & Meyer, 2008). Like Maslow, Rogers (1961) believed that human beings are always striving to fulfil their innate capacities and capabilities and to become everything that their genetic potential allows them to become. This striving for fulfilment is called the self-actualizing tendency. An important tool in human self-actualization is the development of an image of oneself, or the self-concept. The self-concept is based on what people are told by others and how one's sense of self is reflected in the words and actions of important people in one's life, such as parents, siblings, co-workers, friends and teachers. According to the psychology glossary at *alleydog.com* (n.d.), there are many different theories and definitions of 'self' among professional psychologists, but many agree that the 'self' consists of a person's conscious and unconscious aspects, their personality, cognition or thoughts and feelings. All these traits or aspects combine together into the person's core identity. Other synonyms for 'self' are soul, ego, personality or individual. According to the free encyclopedia *Wikipedia* (n.d.), the psychology of self is the study of either the cognitive, conative or affective representation of one's identity or the subject of experience. The earliest formulation of the self in modern psychology is derived from the distinction between the self as *I*, the subjective knower, and the self as *Me*, the object that is known (James, 1891).

5.3.2 Self in Indian Perspective

The concept of self in Indian philosophy is expressed through two different meanings. First, the self as 'aham'/'ahankara', and the other, self as *'atma'*. As far as the field of psychology and present scientific views are concerned, here, the first type of meaning of self as 'aham'/'ahankara' or the feeling of 'I' deserves further discussion. Swami Shivananda (2005) in his book *Manojay* explains that there are three types of the feeling of self:

'Saatvika Ahankara': To feel as I am Brahma.

'Rajsika Ahankara': To feel like I am a king, or intelligent.

'Taamsika Ahankara': To feel I am fool or know nothing.

According to Indian philosophy, the root cause of all troubles is 'ahankara' (feeling of self). Moreover, the aim of all Gyan, Karma and Bhakti Yoga is to be free from 'ahankara' or this feeling of self. Swami Shivananda Ji further describes ahankara as twofold:

'Sthool Ahankara': To feel oneself as a body.

'Sooksma Ahankara': To have this feeling of 'ahankara' about any theory or school.

All the philosophy, religion, knowledge, science, logic and thoughts of the world are concerned with two questions: Here in the world, does a supreme soul or god exist? Or, is the ultimate truth only the observable world? These thoughts lead towards two paths:

1. **Materialism** (scientific thinking)
2. **Spiritualism** (the ultimate truth).

If we have a look at the modern scientific approach, we observe that it has not been able to successfully narrate the evolution of creatures or to describe the world acceptably, because of many incidences failing in this approach. That is why it is well said: *where science ends his thinking, spirituality starts there.*

Spirituality is not only a kind of knowledge, but also a way of life, which we pursue through our religion (duty). Now, this question arises: What is the duty of each person? According to Indian philosophy, there are four types of duty that a human being is compelled to do, since the beginning of our existence:

1. Education (taking and giving).
2. Administering (or to be the part of).
3. Trade.
4. Service (in trade).

As it is said in the *Bhagvad Gita* by Lord Shree Krishna:

> चातुर्वर्ण्यं मया सृष्टं गुणकर्मविभागशः ।
> Chaturvarnayam maya srustam gunkarmvibhagsah.
> तस्य कर्तारमपि मां विद्धयकर्तारमव्ययम् ।।
> Tasya kartarmapi maa vidhyakartarmvyayam.
>
> The four orders of society (viz., the Brahmana, the Ksatriya, the Vaisya and the Sudra) were created by me, classifying them according to the 'Gunas' predominant in each and apportioning corresponding duties to them; though the originator of this creation, know me, the Immortal Lord, to be a non-doer.
>
> *Bhagvad Gita*, 4/13

In all the four kinds, people feel natural and able to do the duty they can do without any material greed. They place spiritual benefit as superior to material benefit, to gain the actual benefits of health, wealth and spirituality. Now the question arises, if people will do their duty without any hope of material result, how can they prosper in their lives? The answer is that when individuals do their duty with 'niskaam bhav' (without hoping for beneficial results), first they will never be mentally stressed and will be free from various mental and physical diseases, and second, because they are doing their duty, they will never lack financial security and can live their lives without any fear or deprivation. Therefore, Shree Krishna obliged Arjuna to do his duty without any hesitation because it was to achieve his earthly (as in name, fame and state) and spiritual (as in ultimate truth) purposes.

> स्वधर्मपि चावेक्ष्य न विकम्पितुमर्हसि ।
> Swadharmapi chavechhya na vikampitumarhasi.
> धर्म्याद्धि युद्धाच्छ्रेयोऽन्यत्क्षत्रियस्य न विद्यते ।।
> Dharmyaddhi yudhachhreyonyatksatriyasya na vidhyate.
>
> Besides, considering your own duty too you should not waver, for there is nothing more welcome for a man of the warrior class than a righteous war.
>
> *Bhagvad Gita*, 2/31

After taking a brief view of some relevant literature in Indian psychology, such as *Yoga*, *Upanishads*, *Bhagvad Gita* and *Vedanta*, among others, it could be concluded that there is undoubtedly sufficient material to build theories and practical implications in the field of mental health which may get better outcomes than others. The model of structure and dynamics of personality as shown in this chapter, should be subject to more scientific and academic interest from scholars and students. Mental health research based on Indian psychology might be more scientific and effective in academic, scholastic, and application fields.

References

Ciccarelli, S. K., & Meyer, G. E. (2008). *Psychology.* (South Asian). Dorling Kindersley Pvt. Ltd.

Freud, S. (1957). *The ego and the Id. Translated by Joan Riviere.* The Hogarth Press Ltd.

James, W. (1891). *The principles of psychology.* Harvard University Press.

Palsane, M. N., Bhavsar, S. N., Goswami, R. P., & Evans, G. W. (1986). The concept of stress in the Indian indicators. *Journal of Indian Psychology, 5*, 1–12.

Psychology glossary at *alleydog.com* (n.d.). Retrieved April 4, 2020, from http://www.alleydog.com/glossary/definition.php?term=Self

Rogers, C. (1961). *On becoming a person: A therapist's view of psychotherapy.* Houghton/Mifflin.

Sharma, N. (2014). Cognitive behaviour therapy in perspective of the Bhagwat Gita. *International Journal of Humanities and Social Science Invention, 3*(1), 2319–7722.

Shivananda, S. (2005). *Manojay.* Divya Jeevan Sangh.

Singh, R. H. (1986). Evaluation of some Indian traditional methods of promotion of mental health. *Activitas Nervosa Superior, 28*, 67–69.

Sinha, D. (1990). Concept of psycho-social well-being: Western and Indian perspectives. *NIMHANS Journal, 8*, 1–11.

Wikipedia, The free encyclopedia. (n.d.). Retrieved April 4, 2020, from http://en.wikipedia.org/wiki/Psychology_of_self

Chapter 6
Indian Psychology and Modern Psychology

6.1 What Is Indian Psychology?

Indian philosophy is one of the oldest studies in the world and is claimed and accepted by many Western and Eastern scholars, as *Rigveda* is one of the oldest complete religious texts (Dutt, 2006). In the form of texts such as the Vedas, Upanishads, Bhagvad Gita, Purana, Mahabharata, Ramayana and many more, there are many 'Granthas' (Books) proving its authenticity. Not only relevant in psychology and the social sciences, Indian philosophy includes all sides of life, ethics, science and so on. As far as psychology and concepts of mental health are concerned, there is ample material in Indian psychology to consider. Before moving on to a short history of Indian psychology, we should first discuss what Indian psychology is, and outline its subject matter.

Indian psychology is an integrative strategy that joins together spirituality and science. This psychological school is created out of the customs of standard, modern psychology blended with the lessons of old Indian texts and practices. The old texts address consciousness, matter, reality and knowledge of typical human inquiries. The old practices, likewise, maintain free limits on their theories: religion, philosophy and psychology are all consolidated into one. This interdisciplinary strategy is the primary allure of this school today. Indian psychologists utilize knowledge on consciousness ('chetna') as an extension between the mind and the outer world, drawing on the lessons of Buddhism, Hinduism and the Vedas (McKeithen, n.d.).

As it was noted before, Indian psychology plays the role of a bridge between spirituality and science. In general, there are pieces of evidence in Indian psychology (philosophy) of all the theories whether old or modern psychology, mainly spirituality, consciousness, matter, reality and typical human questions. Besides this, Indian psychology includes most of the modern psychological aspects of affect, behaviour and cognition (ABC). Psychoanalytic views, humanistic views and other schools have their roots in Indian psychology, which will be discussed later. Indian psychology means the study of psychological concepts in old Indian philosophy, and therefore, it is sometimes studied as Hindu psychology (Akhilananda, 1948). Indian psychology

N. Pant, *Spirituality, Mental Health and Quality of Life*,
https://doi.org/10.1007/978-981-99-2703-6_6

does not mean the psychology research done by Indian researchers in Indian society, or the psychology taught in Indian universities (Cornelissen et al., 2014) (Table 6.1).

To know the concept of Indian psychology well, we should understand that the colonial period in India has not only affected Indian politico-economic conditions, but all areas of society. One such effect has been on the education system, which we are still seeing after so many years of independence. The Western knowledge system remains a major focus of study, in spite of there being such well-established, authentic Indian knowledge systems as Indian philosophy, Yoga, and the Upanishads, Vedas and so forth. Indian psychology has major subject matter in all indigenous psychologies, and that is why they almost seem to be equated with each other. There are many researchers like Durganand Sinha, Janak Pandey, H. G. Singh and Girishwar Misra among others, who have worked on the concept of Indian psychology and given a boost to the subject in its starting phase. Indigenous psychology includes all the traditional approaches of different cultures, or on a cross-cultural basis, in different countries of the world. We see the emphasis of indigenous psychology on relating psychological study, research and application to the native sociocultural context and on developing indigenous concepts, methods, theories and cross-cultural research (Rao & Paranjpe, 2016). Indian psychology, on one hand, has roots in the traditional knowledge sources of India, but, on the other hand, is linked to cultures far beyond its borders, such as in the form of psychoanalysis, CBT, mental health, social psychology and so forth. Thus, Indian psychology is a composite of traditional, modern and

Table 6.1 Characteristics/major fields of Indian psychology

Traditional fields	Modern fields/possibilities
1. Study of soul/'manas'	1. Diagnosis & classification of mental disorders
2. Behavioural knowledge system	2. Positive/transpersonal/para psychology
3. Interpretation of super normal elements	3. Mental health
4. Psychophysical ('mano-daihik')	4. Psychoanalysis
5. Various levels of consciousness ('chetna')	5. Humanistic psychology
6. 'Pancha Koshas': 'Annamya Kosha', 'Pranmaya Kosha', 'Manomaya Kosha', 'Vigyanmaya Kosha', 'Anandamaya Kosha'	6. Values
7. Types of body ('shareer'): 'sthool', 'sooksma', 'karan'	7. Personality
8. Spiritual and religious psychology	8. Cognitive psychology
9. Structure & dynamics of personality: 'gyanndri', 'karmendri', 'manas', 'buddhi', 'atman' etc	9. Emotion
10. Branch of Indian philosophy	10. Spirituality as well as its applications such as meditation etc
	11. Yoga and Ayurveda
	12. Studies of spiritual figures and their legacies

evergreen knowledge sources in the field of psychology. Where unanimous knowledge systems are needed for theory development in the field of psychology, Indian psychology could be used as a major contributor, in spiritual, positive, indigenous, abnormal, clinical and other fields of psychology (Rao & Paranjpe, 2016).

6.1.1 A Short History of Indian Psychology

Here, it is necessary to look at the scholars who have drawn the modern psychologists' attention to the ideas of Indian psychology. In 1910, the term 'Indian psychology' was first used by Sri Aurobindo in one of his writings on education. But the first published work on Indian psychology was completed in 1933 by Jadunath Sinha, with his work, *Indian Psychology: Cognition* (Salagame, 2013). Indian psychology encompasses all indigenous psychological study and research conducted in India from the dawn of time to the present. These developing scholarly and scientific disciplines of psychology are known as Indian psychology. Psychologists working in this area are recovering psychological notions inherent in indigenous Indian religious and spiritual traditions and philosophies and articulating them in psychological language that allows for more psychological investigation and application. Indian psychology does not necessarily imply psychology of the Indian people or psychology taught in Indian universities. Psychologists who have been encouraging or leading recently expanding engagement in this discipline are referred to as members of the Indian psychology movement (Dalal, n.d.).

The subject of Indian psychology gained consideration after the Manifesto on Indian psychology was held in 2002 by many leading psychologists, gathered in Pondicherry, India, and driven by K. Ramakrishna Rao, Girishwar Misra, and others (Matthijs, 2002). Psychologists in this field created insightful and logical contributions that incorporated reading material, a handbook, a few other altered volumes, a diary of exceptional issue, and an assortment of different books and diary articles. Subjects tended to by Indian psychology exploration have included originations pertinent to values, consciousness, personality, cognition, perception, emotion, creativity, education and spirituality as well as applications like meditation, yoga, and ayurveda, and contextual analyses of conspicuous profound figures and their heritages.

During and after British colonial period there were many changes and developments in psychology as a study subject in Indian universities (Dalal, n.d.):

- **1915**: The modern period of Indian psychology began in the Department of Philosophy at the University of Calcutta.
- **1916**: The University of Calcutta established the first Department of Psychology.
- **1922**: The Indian Psychoanalytical Association was founded by Professor Bose.
- **1938**: The Department of Applied Psychology was established.

- **1986**: Durganand Sinha in his book *Psychology in a Third World Country: The Indian Experience*, published in 1986, traces the history of modern psychology as a social science in India in four phases.

The modern period of Indian psychology began in the Department of Philosophy at the University of Calcutta in 1915, where the first course on Experimental Psychology was started and the first psychology laboratory was established. The University of Calcutta also started the first Department of Psychology in 1916 and the Department of Applied Psychology in 1938. Modern experimental psychology was introduced at the University of Calcutta by the Indian psychologist Dr. N. N. Sengupta, who was trained in America in the experimental tradition of Wundt and was greatly influenced by this. Professor Girindra Shekhar Bose was trained in Freud's psychoanalysis; a field that influenced the early development of psychology in India. The Indian Psychoanalytical Association was founded by Professor Bose in 1922 (Rao & Paranjpe, 2016). Early centres of teaching and research in psychology started in Mysore University and Patna University. From the beginning, psychology developed as a strong discipline in India. Now there are many centres of psychology teaching, research and application.

Durganand Sinha, in his book *Psychology in a Third World Country: The Indian Experience* published in 1986, traces the history of modern psychology as a social science in India in four phases. According to him, the *first phase* was up until India's attainment of independence, when there was a lot of emphasis on experimental, psychoanalytical and psychological test research, which reflected the contribution of Western countries in the development of psychology. The *second phase* was the phase after independence and was the start of the identity crisis for the country, and for the subject psychology as well. The *third phase*, from then until 1960, was a time of expansion in various branches of psychology in India. In this phase, Indian psychologists wanted to integrate Western psychology with Indian contexts for Indian identity. They made such an effort to understand Indian conditions through Western ideas. Nevertheless, psychology in India became meaningful to Indian society after 1960 through problem-focused research. Psychologists started paying more attention to the problems of Indian society. Further, an over-reliance on Western psychology began to be felt in its social context. Critical psychologists emphasized the importance of research that was relevant to the current circumstances (Mathew, n.d.). Indigenous psychology emerged in the late 1970s as the *fourth stage*, due to the discovery of a new identity of psychology in India. Apart from rejecting the Western framework, Indian psychologists stressed the need to develop an understanding that is based on socially and culturally meaningful frameworks. This trend was reflected in the efforts that led to the development of approaches based on traditional Indian psychology, which we drew from ancient texts and scriptures. Thus, this phase is characterized by the development of indigenous psychology, which originated from the Indian cultural context, was meaningful to Indian psychology and society and was based on Indian traditional knowledge (Rao, 2008). Now these developments are happening continuously. Psychology in India is making a significant contribution to the field of psychology in the world.

As is well known, Wilhelm Wundt established a first laboratory of psychology in Leipzig, Germany in 1879. On a philosophical and Indian basis, the subject of Indian psychology or philosophy as an academic discipline is not a recent phenomenon. In West Bengal B. N. Seal is reported to have established a psychological laboratory in 1905. The first university department of psychology was established at the University of Calcutta more than 100 years ago in 1915 (Rao & Paranjpe, 2016). N. N. Sengupta was the first head of the Department of Psychology at the University of Calcutta. Sengupta received his training under Hugo Munsterberg at Harvard University, and, as it is known, Munsterberg was the proposer of Applied Psychology. During this time and after, many Indian psychologists were trained and received their degrees in the subject from abroad. As per Misra (2011), psychology in India remains an extension of the Euro-American tradition and continues with Western concepts and methods. However, currently a shift in paradigm is occurring because of the impact of Indian philosophy throughout the world.

Besides this, other Indian psychologists such as Maharishi Mahesh Yogi and Sri Aurbindo, among others, are the eminent proposers of Indian psychology. Maharishi Mahesh Yogi created the concept of Vedic psychology (Bhawuk, 2011) with his meditation techniques and Prasad (1995) showed that mysticism is a corollary to scientific investigation. Sinha (1933) attempted to study the concept of Hindu psychology and was the first proposer of it, and he proposed Indian psychology to be focused basically on introspection and observation. Now psychology in India is being applied in many professional fields. Psychologists are not only working with children with specific problems they are also being appointed as clinical psychologists in hospitals, in corporate organizations like human resources development departments and advertising departments, in sports directorates, the development sector and information technology industries.

6.2 Mahabharata, Bhagvad Gita and Psychology

There are many examples of psychological thoughts in the Mahabharata as shown by the character Shree Krishna. For example, putting an iron idol in front of Dhirstrarashtra to allow Bheema's escape from the aggressive and vengeful thoughts of Dhristrarastra, providing Arjuna with mental support and knowledge while in his depressive phase, as well as many other examples which demonstrate the psychological thought processes of Shree Krishna. The Bhagvad Gita is a 700-verse, 18-chapter dialogue between Shree Krishna and Arjuna, and is part of the epic Mahabharata's Bhisma Parva. Consisting of many spiritual meanings and other fundamental life questions and guidance, the Bhagvad Gita includes many psychological thoughts, too. If one looks at the Mahabharata from a psychological point of view, the character of Shree Krishna is full of psychological instances, such as delivering 'gita gyan' (knowledge) like a counsellor in life situations (Sharma, 2014a), which provides evidence of psychoanalytic thoughts and notions of mental processes.

The original form of the Bhagvad Gita is in Sanskrit and has merely 700 verses ('shlokas'). To interpret it from the perspectives of life, philosophy of life, truth of life and mystery of life, many 'acharyas' (scholars), have made commentaries ('bhasyas') on it. To explain the original verses of the Bhagvad Gita there are many commentaries by Indian saints/scholars, who are famed for their various 'bhasyas' on Gita:

1. **Adi Saṅkara**: The oldest and most influential surviving commentary was given by Adi Shankaracharya, who interprets the Gita in a *non-dualistic* tradition ('Advaita Vedanta').
2. **Ramanuja** disagreed with Adi Shankara's interpretation of the Gita as a text on non-dualism (Self and Brahman are identical), and instead interpreted it as a form of *dualistic* and *qualified monism* philosophy ('Vishishtadvaita').
3. **Madhva**, a commentator of the Dvaita Vedanta School, wrote a commentary on the Bhagavad Gita, which exemplifies the thinking of the *dualist school* (Dvaita Vedanta).
4. **Vallabha**, the proponent of 'Suddhadvaita' or *pure non-dualism*, wrote a commentary on the Gita: the *Sattvadipika.*
5. **Gaudiya Vaishnava**: Chaitanya Mahaprabhu's commentaries on various parts of the Gita are in the Gaudiya Vaishnavism Bhakti ('*Achintya Bhedabheda*').

These are all considered the core paradigms of Indian philosophy (Table 6.2).

6.2.1 Psychological Thoughts in the Bhagvad Gita

The Bhagvad Gita has been found to have significant effect on life situations and efficacy, not only in research review studies but also in empirical studies. Dabas and Singh (2018) studied Indian and Western positive approaches and compared their efficacy for students. For this study, three groups were created. Group 1 was the control group that received the regular course of study followed by schools in the area, Group 2 was given an intervention based on Indian scriptures, mainly the Bhagavad Gita, and Group 3 was given an intervention based on Western positive psychology. Results indicated that the increase in scores for all three variables (hope, optimism and resilience) for the Indian intervention was statistically significant. They concluded that Indian interventions consisted of profound thoughts and mantras that the students could relate to and easily incorporate into most life situations, while it was felt that the positive psychology interventions required more time and expertise for effective implementation.

The Bhagavad Gita reflects the philosophy of 'karma', 'bhakti' and 'gyan yoga' as Krishna's solution to Arjuna's problem is comprehensive, involving the behaviooral ('karma yoga'), the emotional ('bhakti yoga') and the intellectual ('gyan yoga') (Dhakad, 2018). If we view the Bhagvad Gita from a psychological point of view, we find many similar concepts in both psychology and the Gita. For instance (as explored in Chap. 5 also), the major cause of the all the physical problems is the

Table 6.2 Bhagvad Gita and various Yogas in chapters

Chapter	Title (Philosophy & Indian Psychology behind the chapter)	Verses
1.	**'Sainya Darshan'** (सैन्य दर्शन): The first chapter has been translated under a variety of names, including 'Prathama Adhyaya', 'The Distress of Arjuna', 'The War Within', and 'Arjuna's Sorrow'	47
2.	**'Sankhya Yoga'** (सांख्य योग): The chapter is titled 'Sankhya Yoga', 'The Book of Doctrines', 'Self-Realization', or 'The Yoga of Knowledge' (philosophy) by translators, commentators or 'bhasyakaars'	72
3.	**'Karma Yoga'** (कर्म योग): The chapter is titled 'Karma Yoga', 'Virtue in Work', 'Selfless Service', or 'The Yoga of Action' by commentators	43
4.	**'Gyan Yoga'** (ज्ञान योग): 'Jna-Karma-Sanyasa Yoga', 'The Religion of Knowledge', 'Wisdom in Action', or 'The Yoga of Renunciation of Action via Knowledge' are the titles given to the fourth chapter by 'bhasyakaars'	42
5.	**'Karma-Sanyasa Yoga'** (कर्मसंन्यास योग): This chapter is titled 'Karma-Sanyasa Yoga', 'Religion through Renouncing Fruits of Works', 'Renounce and Rejoice', or 'The Yoga of Renunciation' by commentators	29
6.	**'Dhyan Yoga'** (ध्यान योग): The sixth chapter is titled 'Dhyana Yoga', 'Religion through Self-Restraint', 'The Practice of Meditation', or 'The Yoga of Meditation', according to the interpreters	47
7.	**'Vigyan Yoga'** (विज्ञान योग): This chapter is titled 'Jnana-Vijnana Yoga', 'Religion by Discernment', 'Wisdom from Realization', or 'The Yoga of Knowledge and Judgement 'by commentators	30
8.	**'Aksara-ParaBrahma Yoga'** (तारकब्रह्म योग): The chapter is titled 'Aksara-Brahma Yoga' and is also known as 'Religion through Devotion to the One Supreme God', 'The Yoga of the Imperishable Brahman', or 'The Yoga of the Eternal Godhead'	28
9.	**"Raja-Vidya-Raja-Guhya Yoga"** (राजगुह्य योग): The ninth chapter is titled "Raja-Vidya-Raja-Guhya Yoga', also known as 'The Royal Path' or 'The Yoga of Sovereign Science and Sovereign Secret', or 'Religion by the Kingly Knowledge and the Kingly Mystery'	34
10.	**'Vibhuti-Vistara Yoga'** (विभूति योग): The chapter is titled 'Vibhuti-Vistara-Yoga', 'Religion by the Heavenly Perfections', 'Divine Splendour', or 'The Yoga of Divine Manifestations', according to the interpreters	42
11.	**'Viswarupa-Darsana Yoga'** (विश्वरूप-दर्शन योग): The chapter is titled 'Vishvarupa-Darshana Yoga', 'The Manifestation of the One and Manifold', 'The Cosmic Vision', or 'The Yoga of the Vision of the Cosmic Form' by the translators	55
12.	**'Bhakti Yoga'** (भक्ति योग): The chapter is titled 'Bhakti Yoga', 'The Religion of Faith', 'The Way of Love', or 'The Yoga of Devotion' by the interpreters	20
13.	**'Ksetra-Ksetrajna Vibhaga Yoga'** (प्रकृति-पुरुष-विभाग योग): This chapter is titled 'The Yoga of Difference between the Field and Field-Knower', 'Ksetra-Ksetrajna Vibhaga Yoga', 'Religion through Separation of Matter and Spirit', or 'The Field and the Knower' by different interpreters	34

(continued)

Table 6.2 (continued)

Chapter	Title (Philosophy & Indian Psychology behind the chapter)	Verses
14.	**'Gunatraya-Vibhaga Yoga'** (गुणत्रय-विभाग योग): The fourteenth chapter is referred to as 'Gunatraya-Vibhaga Yoga', 'Religion by Separation from the Qualities', 'The Forces of Evolution', or 'The Yoga of the Division of Three Gunas' by the various commentators	27
15.	**'Purushottama-Prapti Yoga'** (पुरुषोत्तम योग): 'Purushottama Yoga', is also known as 'The Yoga of the Supreme Purusha', 'The Religion through Attaining the Supreme Krishna', or 'The Supreme Self', in different translations of this chapter	20
16.	**'Daivasura-Sampad-Vibhaga Yoga'** (दैवासुरसम्पद योग): The chapter is titled 'Daivasura-Sampad-Vibhaga Yoga', 'The Separation of the Divine and Undivine', 'Two Paths', or 'The Yoga of the Division between the Divine and the Demonic' by the commentators	24
17.	**'Shraddhatraya-Vibhaga Yoga'** (श्रद्धात्रय विभाग योग): The chapter is titled 'Shraddhatraya-Vibhaga Yoga' by the translators, which can also be rendered as 'The Yoga of the Threefold Faith', 'The Power of Faith', or 'Religion by the Threefold Kinds of Faith'	28
18.	**'Moksha-Sanyasa Yoga'** (मोक्ष योग): The chapter is titled' Moksha-Sanyasa Yoga', 'Religion of Deliverance and Renunciation', 'Freedom and Renunciation', or 'The Yoga of Liberation and Renunciation' by the commentators	78
	Total	700

mental illness as it is found in modern and ancient studies. Frequent occurring and observable problem of current time is faulty life style and aimless life. Mentality of the society has become to get economy and have material fun. That is why Bhagwan Shree Krishna in Bhagvad Gita told:

ध्यायतो विष्यान्पुन्सः संगस्तेषूप्जायते
Dhyayato vishyanpunsah sangasteshoopjaayate,

संगात्संजायते कामः कामात्क्रोधोभिजायते
Sangaatsanjaayate kaamah kaamaatkrodhobhijayate.

(*Essence: The origination of diseases is only due to lust of human being towards life and physical world. Diseases originates because of faulty life style and perceptions*)

Bhagvad Gita *2/62*

6.2.1.1 The Bhagvad Gita and Psychotherapies

Many psychotherapy themes can be found in the discussion between Arjuna and Shree Krishna. Arjuna displayed a form of twisted thinking at the start of the conflict. Shree Krishna assists with this through a psychological technique known as Cognitive Behavioural Therapy (CBT) (Sharma, 2014a). The Bhagavad Gita contains much CBT material. Despite being the greatest warrior of his day, Arjuna suffered from anxiety, grief, guilt, fear and depression, and Krishna worked as a therapist for him. Much of the Bhagvad Gita can be viewed as a collection of cognitive behavioural treatment sessions. Through his therapy, the Krishna changed Arjuna's warped thoughts, emotions and behaviour, and Arjuna expressed respect and devotion to his therapist. Arjuna's anguish was caused by his fear of sin and the loss of loved ones, but the Krishna dispelled his worries by teaching him about 'Karma' (activity), 'Yoga' (skill in action), 'Nirvana' (detachment) and the eternal nature of the soul. If the patient is cooperative, CBT can be made easier (Sharma, 2014b).

In this way, the Bhagvad Gita draws parallels between the Gita's teachings and a variety of psychotherapy themes, including CBT, grief emancipation, role transition, self-esteem and motivation enhancement, as well as interpersonal and supportive psychotherapies (Bhatia et al., 2013). Other psychotherapies found in Bhagvad Gita include psychodynamic psychotherapy and mindfulness.

6.2.1.2 The Bhagvad Gita and Motivation

The way Arjuna is inspired to achieve his goal in the Gita not only inspires people today, but also gives a way for people to move forward in the future and directs them to take action. People also enter the same state of mind that Arjuna did prior to the conflict. When confronted with such conditions, people may despair and, after sinking deeper into the abyss of disappointment, they may resort to extreme measures such as suicide (Dhakad, 2018). Shree Krishna's everlasting voice gives hope to everyone who is suffering from mental illness and weaknesses when he says:

> क्लैब्यं मा स्म गमः पार्थ नैतत्त्वय्युपपद्यते। क्षुद्रं हृदयदौर्बल्यं त्यक्त्वोत्तिष्ठ परन्तप।।
>
> It does not befit you to yield to this unmanliness. Give up such petty weakness of heart and arise, O vanquisher of enemies.
>
> Bhagvad Gita *2/3*

6.2.1.3 The Bhagvad Gita and Adjustment

According to modern psychologists, adjustment is a process by which humans and animals balance their needs and the situations that affect their fulfilment. This means that when individuals are unable to meet their natural needs, they gradually compromise with unpleasant situations (Dhakad, 2018). In psychology, this compromise is referred to as adjustment. The word 'adjustment' is used in the Bhagvad Gita to refer to the art of life. Adjustment is the state of equanimity, as stated in the following 'sloka':

> इहैव तैर्जितः सर्गो येषां साम्ये स्थितं मनः। निर्दोषं हि समं ब्रह्म तस्माद् ब्रह्मणि ते स्थिताः।।
>
> Those whose minds are established in equality of vision conquer the cycle of birth and death in this very life. They possess the flawless qualities of God and are therefore seated in the Absolute Truth.
>
> Bhagvad Gita *5/19*

In the second chapter, Shree Krishna's sermon on 'isthitpragyata' (balanced mind) laid the groundwork for Arjuna's mental stability. Arjuna says, at this point, that to pacify a restless, turbulent, and rebellious mind is even more difficult than controlling the wind. Shree Krishna, on the other hand, rouses him. After being inspired, Arjuna's spirit soared.

6.3 Yoga

Yoga Sutra is the famous creation of Maharishee Patanjali. This is Sri Aurobindo, who brought the attention of psychology and modern science to scientific perspective of yoga as *Integral Yoga* which means *Satchidananda*, and is called *Supramental Yoga* too. Integral yoga includes six branches of traditional yoga: Hatha Yoga, Raja Yoga, Bhakti Yoga, Karma Yoga, Gyan Yoga and Japa Yoga. In the early 1900s, Sri Aurobindo founded Integral Yoga, which he defined as:

> a path of integral seeking of the Divine by which all that we are is liberated in the end from Ignorance and its undivine formations into a truth beyond the Mind, a truth not only of highest spiritual status but of a dynamic spiritual self-manifestation in the universe.

In his opus *The Synthesis of Yoga*, Sri Aurobindo explores the nature and practice of Integral Yoga (Aurobindo, 1999). His Integral Yoga is the synthesis of yoga, as the term suggests, designed to integrate the pathways of Karma, Gyana and Bhakti Yoga as taught in the Bhagvad Gita.

6.3.1 Psychological Thoughts in Yoga

Yoga is a whole way of living for self-transformation, spiritual development and becoming a more refined human being. Yoga, as a spiritual discipline, assists in going beyond modern psychology's current understanding of mind to investigate, experience and expand the spectrum of our psychical potentialities and awareness. Much early study on yoga was conducted in different circumstances from the perspective of modern psychology. It was first studied as a method for mastering what was previously referred to as the involuntary nervous system or autonomic nervous system. Many other techniques like biofeedback are related with the Yoga theories developed by Maharishi Patanjali. Second, research which was conducted to better understand the brain-behaviour relationship has led some experts to wonder if practising yoga has similar impacts on the brain and nervous system in humans. Third, research on Maharshi Mahesh Yogi's Transcendental Meditation at Harvard University sparked worldwide interest in its potential to promote calmness. The term 'relaxation response' was coined by Benson and his colleagues to characterize the numerous physiological and psychological changes observed in Transcendental Meditation practitioners (Salagame, 2002). This research opened up a lot of possibilities for using meditative practices in clinical settings. Fourth, researchers who were interested in the study of consciousness, used yoga techniques to induce altered states of consciousness. Meditation research has evolved in two key areas, namely as a 'self-regulation approach' and as an 'altered states of consciousness'. Thus, throughout the last five decades, scientific research on yoga has developed to uncover its potential as a clinical intervention for lowering anxiety or stress, depression and other mental health issues, as well as to investigate its physiological and psychological impacts. The nature and process of meditation experiences have been studied using psychodynamic, behavioural, cognitive, humanistic-existential and transpersonal approaches.

Much of what Patanjali has said, or what the Upanishads or spiritual teachings of any other tradition have to say, cannot be comprehended without a new paradigm. In truth, ancient philosophers in India did not place much emphasis on mental activities and processes, to the point where there was no separate branch of knowledge dedicated to the study of the mind. They were more interested in the soul's emancipation. The mind was discussed from the perspective of liberation, and, therefore, it was included in what is known in India as 'Adhytma', or spiritual quest. The ultimate goal of yoga, according to the 'Samkhya' paradigm, is to distinguish the two and realize 'Purusha', the principle of consciousness. 'Prakruti' is divided into three 'gunas' in this paradigm: 'sattva', 'rajas' and 'tamas'. Many people translate these three as the primal essences or principles of light, energy and inertia, which give rise to both mental and physical phenomena in varied quantities. Material phenomena are dominated by 'tamas', while mental experiences are predominantly dominated by 'sattva'. As a result, mind-matter is seens as a continuum rather than categories as defined by Western intellectual traditions (Salagame, 2010a). While Indian traditions recognize the existence of a duality between pure consciousness and matter, the Western tradition does not.

Most transpersonalists fail to distinguish between 'transpersonal' and 'transcendental', so attempts to approach yoga as transpersonal psychology do not meet the requirement of its original purposes (Salagame, 2010b). The definition of Yoga by Patanjali serves as an example of this. Yoga is defined by Patanjali as 'chitta vrtti nirodhah', which implies the cessation of all mental activity, including ordinary and non-ordinary cognition, affect and volition. This viewpoint can be conveyed more clearly with the help of a line (seventh verse) from the Mandkya Upanishad. This seventh verse clarifies all three states: 'jagrat' (waking), 'swapna' (dream), and 'sushupti' (sleep). These are mental states (as in awake and dreaming) or their absence (as in sleep), but not pure consciousness. Because it had learned from modern psychology literature that altered states of consciousness refer to changes in mental functioning that are fundamentally different from typical waking states, furthermore, the three states and the concept of atman had the Gestalt impact of figure-ground reversal (Salagame, 1988, 2002).

Yoga has been seen by some researchers as biofeedback and as a practical technique of achieving mental calm, and the encouraging findings of the studies demonstrate the interdependence of the body and the mind (Manickam, 2005). In reality, there are many different forms of yoga. Yoga's literal meanings, then again, are:

Union with the ultimate truth, union with God, or union with pure consciousness. Yoga essentially has a spiritual component, and, when all of its components are practised together, not only the physical 'asanas' or poses, something changes that results in an integrative transformation. Different dimensions, including the physical, psychophysical, cerebral, intellectual and spiritual, all experience transformation. This goal has been lived and accomplished at various levels by wise individuals as well as by highly determined individuals. Not just individuals who suffer from various illnesses but also those who are working toward a greater condition of self-realization experience the transition (Manickam, 2005).

6.3.1.1 Psychophysiology

The Yoga Sutra of Patanjali and Kundalini Yoga can both aid in the development of yoga as a psychology of transformation. Most recent studies have concentrated on specific types of yoga, such as Hatha Yoga, Raja Yoga and Kundalini Yoga, rather than on yoga as an end state, 'Samatvam', and 'Stithapragya'. Many mystics testify for their experienced actuality, despite the fact that current anatomical procedures cannot find them through laboratory dissection of the human body. The pineal gland, according to Roney Dougal in her studies done in 1999, is the physical location of the 'Agya' chakra, which is regarded as the psychic centre of our existence in yogic tradition (as reported by Salagame, 2010a). She delves into the yogic concept of the 'Agya' chakra as the command chakra, which oversees the functioning of the other chakra centres. She points out that melatonin is frequently mentioned as the 'off switch' for the endocrine gland's hormone secretion, operating in tandem with the pituitary gland, which is thought to be the 'on switch.' The thyroid of 'vishuddhi', the breasts of 'anhatha', the adrenals of 'manipura', and the gonads of 'swadhistna' and 'muldhra' are all physical aspects of the 'Agya' chakra, according to her. These endocrine glands are all located at distinct chakras, and their functions correspond to those described in traditional chakra descriptions. She claims that the endocrine system represents the physiological element of the yogic spiritual tradition of the chakras, and that the autonomic nervous system is equivalent to the yogic 'Nadis' (Salagame, 2010a). In Indian tradition, three sorts of bodies are distinguished: 'Sthool' (gross), 'sooksma' (subtle), and 'karan' (causal), with Kundalini Shakti predominantly based in the latter two, with secondary manifestations in the first. Many researchers dismiss indigenous perspectives on such events in favour of reductionism.

Understanding the relevance and scope of psychophysiology or somatic psychology advancements is helpful in attempting to establish a synthesis between yoga and Western psychology. It may construct a comparable bridge between psychotherapy and yoga by understanding how somatic psychology connects psychotherapy and somatic bodywork. Yoga psychotherapy is an integrative framework that has a tremendous impact on cultivating wellness with its own language and set of activities (Caplan et al., 2013).

Body consciousness is becoming more widely recognized in the West as an important component of psychological wellbeing (Mehling et al., 2011). Psychophysiology has been demonstrated to be useful in treating anxiety, depression, psychosomatic disorders, PTSD, sexual abuse and other forms of trauma (Berg et al., 2010; Steckler & Young, 2009). Body-based therapies improve self-regulation, develop body awareness, minimize dissociation, promote self-care and pain management abilities and allow the body's intrinsic intelligence to emerge to help complete impulses that may have been blocked during the traumatic event (Lopez, 2011; Price, 2005). There is a broad body of literature on the benefits of physical yoga and contemplative practices for health, happiness and psychological issues for integrating yoga and Western psychology, particularly in light of results in psychophysiology, neuroscience and trauma research. Only a few researchers (Emerson et al., 2009; Van, 2006) have published on how yoga and psychology can link each other, enhancing the effectiveness of each to create an integral model seeking to reduce the effects of psychological trauma.

6.3.1.2 Clinical Psychology

Yoga has been shown to help a variety of psychiatric illnesses, according to the DSM-5 (American Psychiatric Association, 2013) (as reported by Caplan et al., 2013). A yoga practice has been demonstrated to regulate emotions, reduce hyperactivity and impulsivity, increase attention span, feelings of tranquilly and confidence and improve social skills in children with Attention Deficit Hyperactivity Disorder (ADHD).

Stress: Numerous studies have shown that practising yogic 'asanas' physically reduces stress and promotes increased relaxation and regulation on a psychological and neuromuscular level. As per Harvard Health Publications (2009), yoga plays an important role in stress management. Yoga appears to alter stress response systems by lowering perceived stress and anxiety. This, in turn, lowers physiological arousal, lowering heart rate, blood pressure and respiration. Yoga has also been shown to improve heart rate variability, which is a measure of the body's ability to respond to stress more flexibly. Yoga helps to train the body to relax on a muscle level, making it easier to moderate the stress reaction (Serber, 2000). Brisbon and Lowery (2011) discovered that advanced Hatha Yoga practitioners had lower stress levels and a greater sense of being present in the moment than beginners.

Yoga also provides a framework for emotional regulation and a place to practise self-soothing strategies (Harper, 2010). A study by Gootjes et al. (2011) found that yogic meditative techniques aid in good emotion control. There is also evidence that yoga can help traumatized children develop their self-soothing abilities (Spinazzola et al., 2011). Overall, yoga has been proven to enhance stress management at a level comparable to cognitive behavioural therapies, aiding relaxation and mood regulation (Granath, 2006). Breath work has also been shown to improve emotional regulation and heart rate variability by harmonizing the relationship between the sympathetic and parasympathetic nervous systems (Brown & Gerbarg, 2009).

Depression: There are many research studies supporting the relationship of depression and yogic practices. Kinser et al. (2013) discovered that women diagnosed with major depressive disorders, who were allocated to a yoga intervention group, experienced decreased ruminations, improved feelings of closeness and the added benefit of learning a new coping skill. According to Forbes (2008), yoga's ability to relax the nervous system, cultivate present-moment consciousness and release trapped energy in the body aids in the decrease of symptoms linked with affective disorders. The practice of the breath has been demonstrated to be beneficial in the treatment of depression and anxiety in studies. According to Miller (1994), yogic, diaphragmatic breathing improves ego strength, emotional stability, confidence, alertness, and perceived control over one's environment, as well as reducing anxiety, depression, phobic behaviour and psychosomatic disorders. Lalande et al. (2012) looked at how suppressing inner experiences, which can be prompted by traumatic situations, is associated with inhibited breathing, which can exacerbate depression and anxiety. Furthermore, according to Baer (2003), mindfulness-based interventions may be beneficial in the treatment of a variety of conditions, including chronic pain, anxiety, depression, eating disorders, cancer patients, fibromyalgia and psoriasis, with positive results. Weintraub (2004) goes over the many yoga techniques that can be utilized to treat depression in great depth. Her work was based on research as well as her personal experience of using yoga to heal and manage depression.

Caplan et al. (2013) conducted a review of major studies on yoga (including 'asana', breath control, and meditation), somatic psychology and trauma, and discovered that yoga and psychology are complementary to one another, and that their integration aids in the recovery process from psychological trauma. Finally, Caplan et al. (2013) presented the following five perspectives and integration possibilities:

1. **A complete picture of yoga and how this ancient practice can complement modern psychological theory and clinical treatment can assist Western psychologists**. By modulating the stress response and managing emotions, yoga and yogic approaches have been found to alleviate stress and anxiety. They boost emotions of closeness, confidence, attention, body awareness and perceived control over the environment, as well as overall wellbeing and pleasure with life.
2. **As a result of these beneficial effects of yoga, symptoms of a number of DSM-5 diseases, such as ADHD, eating disorders, schizophrenia, and depression, can be reduced**. Many of the concerns associated with PTSD and related symptomology, such as the inability to self-soothe and moderate arousal, fear and dissociation from the body, and continuous stress that draws the individual out of the present and into the trauma, appear to be addressed by the positive advantages.
3. **This integration can benefit Western yoga practitioners by broadening their understanding of yoga to include a psychological component**. This allows for a deeper dive into the practice, focusing on how yoga can alter one's sense of self and increase wellbeing in both formal and everyday yoga practice.
4. **Embodiment**: Human beings have the potential to become fully embodied, meaning that the consciousness and intelligence normally associated with the

mind can awaken across the entire body. Yoga and psychology are combined to assist whole-body awakening by helping people to work through psychological holding patterns, traumas and diseases while also connecting to their bodies and the present moment.

5. **In considering trauma**, the integration of yoga and psychology opens up many possibilities for trauma-sensitive yoga approaches to be developed, explored and implemented.

6.3.1.3 Carl Jung

Jung studied Hinduism and was interested in yoga. Jung recognized that yoga served a higher purpose than keeping the body in shape namely, spiritual alignment. Yoga uses seven separate 'Mandalas', which are symbolic representations of the seven stages of the unconscious mind, to help practitioners grasp the Self (Karani, 2014). For the majority of his career, Jung saw parapsychological events as coming from the collective unconscious rather than supra-physical levels of consciousness that exist independently of the human psyche. As a result, Jung viewed possession states and other dark phenomena as projections from a shadow aspect of self that needed to be psychologically integrated. In contrast, Integral Yoga psychology views adverse forces and the 'Inconscient' as spiritual realities, emphasizing volitional efforts to reject or modify them rather than attempting to explain them as split-off components of a Jungian shadow that must be psychologically worked through.

6.4 Veda and Psychology

6.4.1 Vedic Psychology (Maharishi Mahesh Yogi)

According to Vedic psychology, the mind is divided into layers that range from gross to subtle; from highly active to settled; from concrete to abstract; and from diverse to united (Maharishi Mahesh Yogi, 1972). The action and sense faculties, desire, the thinking mind, the discriminating intellect, feeling and intuition and the individual ego are the levels of mind defined by Mahesh Yogi (Maharishi Mahesh Yogi, 1969). Human development is viewed in the model as a progression from the *dominant level of consciousness* to successively deeper levels of mind: From *senses* (sensorimotor stage) to *desire* (preoperational stage) to *mind* (concrete operational stage) to *intellect* (formal operational stage) to *feeling and intuition* (early post formal, postconventional stage) to *ego* (late post formal, postconventional stage). According to Alexander (2005) the functioning of conscious awareness at each successively deeper intrinsic level of the mind may offer the foundation for each successively greater manifestation of cognitive and personality growth observed by developmental psychologists. Although the ultimate status of the knower or 'I' is always pure consciousness (Maharishi Mahesh Yogi, 1969), awareness becomes localized or conditioned by active mind processes and corresponding nervous system structures in the waking state of consciousness. Human growth, according to Alexander's concept, is a U-shaped function that begins with inward development until transcendental consciousness is achieved, and then moves outward as the attributes of transcendental consciousness are brought into all levels of mind and behaviour (Orme-Johnson, 2000).

Mahesh Yogi's Vedic psychology theory of human development recognizes seven levels of human consciousness, four of which are higher states of consciousness than the three psychophysiologically characterized states of awake, dreaming, and sleeping. According to the assumption, practising the Maharishi Technology of the Unified Field automatically accelerates the development of higher states. The Transcendental Meditation technique is described as a simple, natural mental procedure that allows a person to experience less enthusiastic, progressively refined levels of mental activity and to move beyond all excited states of the mind to the least thrilled state of mental activity, known as transcendental consciousness. There are meditational programmess based in Mahesh Yogi's theories, such as the Transcendental Meditation-Sidhi programme, which incorporates sophisticated mental techniques that improve mind–body coordination and promote the ability to work at the level of transcendental consciousness, speeding up the progression to higher states of consciousness. Because it is the foundation on which all higher phases of growth take place, transcendent consciousness is important to Vedic psychology's theory of seven states of consciousness (Alexander et al., 1987). Some key points of Mahesh Yogi's Vedic psychology are in the following section.

6.4.1.1 Seven States of Human Consciousness

Vedic science's idea of human evolution delineates seven major stages of human consciousness (Alexander et al., 1987; Maharishi Mahesh Yogi, 1972). Each level of consciousness has its own set of physiological correlates and produces different types of knowledge. The first three are universal human experiences (awake, dreaming, and sleeping), while the latter four are higher states. Transcendental consciousness, the fourth state, is crucial to this idea because frequent experience of it cultures the physiology and gives rise to the subsequent states.

The seven states and their associated forms of knowledge are as follows:

1. In a deep state of slumber (sleep) there is no sense of self or environment. There will be no self-referrals.
2. The state of dreaming: Self- or environment-related illusions. Self-referral is extremely rare.
3. The state of awakening: The surface value of the environment and the experience of excited levels of mental activity. The active levels of thinking and perception obfuscate the fundamental essence of the self as transcendental consciousness. Self-referral consciousness is fragmented, and it is seen as a knower, a known, and a knowing process.

4. Transcendental: The state of consciousness with the least amount of excitement, pure consciousness, the source of cognition, and the most basic kind of consciousness. Thought and perception are no longer relevant. The cosmic psyche is a completeness of pure consciousness in which the knower, the known and the act of knowing coincide. Infinity awakens to itself for the first time in the state of self-referral. It is wholeness, aware of itself, devoid of difference, transcendental consciousness beyond the separation of subject and object (Maharishi Mahesh Yogi, 1977).
5. Cosmic: With the various states of waking, dreaming, and deep sleep, the self is permanently preserved. The Self, in its self-referral state of pure consciousness, passively observes daily activities.
6. God Consciousness: Perception of the highest manifest value of or refined cosmic every object, as well as the Self's constant consciousness experience. In this level of consciousness, the value of relative existence has been polished to its highest level. Between the knower's limitless self-referral nature and the boundaries of the objects known, only the finest separation exists.
7. Consistency consciousness is the complete potential of natural law, and it is the full realization of the cosmic psyche. The position of self-referral has been elevated to absolute. Every point in creation contains infinity, and every point in creation is elevated to the limitless state of the self. The Self acting within itself is revealed to be the source of all cosmic life (Alexander & Boyer, 1989).

6.4.1.2 Developmental Theory

Mahesh Yogi's Vedic psychology provides a theory of levels of mind, in addition to the notion of seven states of consciousness, which describes the structural and functional links between consciousness and sensory, cognitive and affective processes (Dillbeck & Alexander, 1989). According to this idea, the human mind has a hierarchical structure with levels of functional depth ranging from gross to subtle, culminating in the transcendental foundation of individual mind, the unified field of consciousness. In order of progressive subtlety and abstraction, Vedic psychology delineates the following components of the individual psyche: (1) the most expressed level, the senses; (2) that which directs attention to the objects of sensations, desire; (3) the active thinking level, referred to as mind; (4) the discriminative processes, referred to as intellect; and (5) the most subtle, integrative function of individuality, the ego. Pure consciousness, the cosmic psyche, lies beneath various levels of the individual mind. According to Maharishi (as reported by Alexander et al., 1987) the levels of mind influence behaviour: Action is carried out through the senses, but it has its origins at the beginning of the thought process. An idea originates at the deepest level of the mind; it is evaluated on the thinking level, where it manifests as a desire. Desire, in turn, manifests as action.

From birth through early adulthood, cognitive development takes place in stages, progressing from more concrete to increasingly abstract or subtle states. The deep structure for the unfoldment of each corresponding higher level of cognitive development may be provided by the progressive enlivenment of each subtler level of mind. Although all levels of mind contribute to the growth of every idea and developmental stage, the deepest levels of mind and the underlying cosmic psyche are usually beyond the conscious range of appreciation and usage. When conscious awareness begins to operate primarily from a deeper level of mind, a matching developmental stage is expected to stabilize (Dillbeck & Alexander, 1989). From birth to adolescence or early adulthood, Piaget identified four basic cognitive-structural stages: (1) the sensorimotor stage, (2) the pre-operational level dominated by immediate impulse and perception, (3) the concrete mental operations stage, and (4) the level of abstract reflective thought, formal operations (Piaget & Inhelder, 1969). The nature and sequence of more sophisticated levels of mind defined by Vedic psychology are: action and the senses, impression and desire, the active thinking mind, and abstract discriminating intellect, respectively, and bear an interesting parallel to the sequential unfoldment of these phases (Dillbeck & Alexander, 1989). Piaget's approach, on the other hand, stops at typical adult conceptual thought and ignores the possibility of postconceptual growth of higher states of consciousness based on understanding of the cosmic psyche at the source of thought.

Unified Field and Cognitive Development: From a developmental standpoint, the Mahesh Yogi's Technology of the Unified Field appears to be as important as language learning for promoting development beyond the sensorimotor and preconceptual levels of early childhood to postconceptual higher states of consciousness (Alexander & Bodeker, 1982). This technique encourages postconceptual growth by allowing the mind to bypass conceptual thinking and directly experience the content-free state of pure consciousness at the root of thought. Conscious awareness grows to function from progressively deeper levels of mind during the Transcendental Meditation process of transcending, promoting comparable psychological growth. According to studies, the unique condition of peaceful awareness induced by the Transcendental Meditation technique effectively neutralizes deep-seated stress, allowing for continued human development (Jevning et al., 1978; Wallace, 1986). There are many research studies to validate and justify the Mahesh Yogi's techniques of Vedic psychology having cognitive developmental effects. According to one study, the Maharishi Technology of the Unified Field speeds up cognitive development in children and unfreezes development that is usually frozen in maturity (Dillbeck & Alexander, 1989). Even after accounting for probable demographic variations between the groups in terms of age, gender and parental socioeconomic background, children participating in the Transcendental Meditation programme scored considerably higher on Piagetian measures of cognitive development than children in the control group. According to cross-sectional and longitudinal studies, the Transcendental Meditation approach may help adolescents and young adults improve moral reasoning. Furthermore, repetition of this strategy has been proven to improve a variety of cognitive functions that generally get fixed in early adulthood. Longitudinal studies have found that Transcendental Meditation practitioners outperform controls on measures of fluid intelligence field independence (Aron et al., 1981; Tjoa, 1975).

These findings show that the Mahesh Yogi's Technology of the Unified Field may be able to not only unfreeze cognitive-structural development, but also reverse age-related losses. As per a study reported in Alexander et al. (1987)'s study, participants of an average age of 81 years were randomly allocated to treatment and no-treatment groups that were identical in external structure and expectation-fostering aspects in another demographic that is often resistant to change: the institutionalized elderly. Learning capacity, cognitive flexibility, systolic blood pressure, mental health and self-rating of behavioural flexibility and ageing all improved the most in the Transcendental Meditation group, despite comparability in pre-test measures and expectations. After three years, the Transcendental Meditation group's survival rate (longevity) was 100 per cent, compared to 76 per cent for the other therapy groups and 62.5 per cent for the other 478 residents of the nursing homes for the elderly.

6.5 Atharva Veda

The abnormalities or classification of mental disorders described in the Indian studies and Atharva Veda can be categorized in a variety of ways. There are many classifications proposed in the Indian perspective. Wig and Singh (1967) introduced the various types of psychosis, and further, J. S. Teja (1971), described psychosis in five parts. Arsh (1999) divided the mental disorders discussed in the Atharva Veda into two categories: severe disturbances such as 'unmaad', and mental process faults such as 'krodh' (anger), 'moh' (attachment), 'shok' (depression), and 'dushswapna' (bad dreams), the same as Tulsidasji suggested in Ramcharitmanas. But Singh (1977)'s name is worth discussing in doing the proper categorization and classification of mental disorders in the Indian perspective. Singh (1977) proposed a more logical taxonomy, dividing the mental diseases described in the Atharva Veda into three categories:

1. **'Gambheer Vikriti' (Severe disorders)**: These are the disorders that are the furthest away from normalcy. 'unmaad' (insanity), 'grahi' (seizure or hysterical fits), 'apasmar' (epilepsy), 'durbhiti' (phobia), 'manovidalita' (schizophrenia), and 'paap-bhaav' and 'heenta' (guilt feeling and inferiority feeling) are some of the terms used.
2. **'Sadharan Vikriti' (Mild disorder)**: This type of disease is characterized by a divergence from normal mental processes. They present in regular conduct, however to a greater extent in pathological behaviour, such as 'krodh' (anger), 'irshya' (jealousy), 'moh' (eroticism), 'duhswapnn' (evil dream) and 'bahya shraap' (compulsive evil suggestion) etc.
3. **Swasthya and Sangathan (Health and integration)**: The following disorders fall under this category: 'buddhi evam smriti vardhan' (intelligence and memory improvement), 'pustikani' or 'aham-urjan' (ego emerging) and 'samansaa sasyani' or 'samajic sangathan' (social integration). Singh focuses on ways to develop one's personality and mental health through positive approaches. These

are concerned with memory and learning enhancements, as well as 'atmabal' or activating the ego integration and harmony inside the individual. It is a unique feature of the Atharva Veda and all other Indian systems that they place a greater emphasis on the pleasant aspects of life rather than the negative aspects of ailments and diseases.

The Atharva Veda method is therapeutic in nature. It is not diagnostic in nature. The sage authors of the Atharva Veda ignored symptoms and diagnosis. At the moment, the two 'Shakhas' available, 'Piplad' and 'Shaunk', deal with the symptoms and diagnosis of mental diseases in a rather vague manner, despite being very rich in therapy.

6.5.1 Psychotherapies

In Atharva Veda, there is no firm and fast division or classification of therapies. For one condition, there are various types of therapies, and for many disorders, there is only one type of therapy. The treatments may not have to be done in that order. Their characteristics, such as Havan-prayer, frequently overlap. Suggestion and re-education are used in all of Atharva Veda's therapies. A broad taxonomy of therapeutic methods for mental diseases is described in the Atharva Veda. The following therapies are the most frequent among them, and therapists use them to help people strengthen their minds and cure diseases. 'Manas Chikitsa': When a therapy is primarily centred on psychological aspects, it is referred to as 'manas chikitsa', or therapy that originates from inside oneself rather than from outside influences. Some examples of 'manas chikitsa' described in the Atharva Veda are: 'Mantra Vidya', 'Sankalpa' (auto-suggestion), 'Sandesh' (suggestion), 'Samvashikaran' (hypnosis), 'Ritualistic Therapy' (drama and demonstration), 'Brahma Kavach' (psychological defensive belief), 'Utarna' (transference), 'Ashwasana' and 'Upchar' (assurance, desensitization, re-education), 'Davaiya Havan Chikitisa' (spiritual prayer with 'havan' and rituals), Tapa/Tyag (penance/sacrifice).

1. **'Mantra Vidya'** (mantra therapy): Mantra is the main technique of 'manas chikitsa'. 'Mantra' is a word that means 'hidden talk'. Mantra, as is well known, is neither a mere letter, or a group of letters with some significance, writes Shashtri (1951). It is the powerful sound body shared by the intense vibrations of the creator's spiritual personality or the seer of mantra. The mantra is a living incarnation of truth and power that has found expression in it through the rishis or yogis who have given it a body. The mantra might be composed of words or single characters organized in a specific order. Mantras can be used in a variety of ways in psychotherapy. They serve various purposes in various ways. The same mantra can be applied to various situations and in various ways. Mantras are also associated with various therapies.
2. **'Sankalpa'** (auto-suggestion): 'Sankalpa' literally means willpower or 'atmabal'. In psychology, it refers to the ego's strength. It's a type of therapy in

which patients attempt to heal themselves. In Atharva Veda, it is declared that the patient is the best physician. It can be utilized for both individual and group treatment. The ego can be made robust and active, and capable of dealing with its challenges, using the 'sankalpa' approach. There can be no psychological personality breakdown with a robust ego.

3. **'Sandesh'** (suggestion): In 'Sankalpa', there is no therapist, and thus, the patients gave themselves advice or suggestions. However, in the case of 'Sandesh', the advice is supplied by a third party, such as a guru, priest or therapist. In "Sandesh', the therapist has a director role, while the patient has a passive position as a follower or a recipient. The practitioner of therapy, or 'manas chikitsak', must be a 'Brahma-gyani', or someone who understands and works with Brahma's energy. The 'chikitsak', according to Arsh (1999), must be serious, truthful, self-controlled and helpful. As a result, practitioners have a greater impact on their patients due to their own mental energy. This can be utilized in 'grahi', 'phobia', 'apasmar', 'pap bhawna', 'krodh', 'irshya', 'moh', 'shrap', 'samansayani', and 'paushtikarni' as a key therapy for mental diseases.
4. **'Samvashikaran'** (hypnosis): This is a unique kind of suggestion. The therapist's personality and mental capacity are the major forces in this advanced effective stage of suggestibility. The therapist may then make other recommendations. Actually, in 'Samvashikaran', the therapist takes control of and directs the patient's mind. 'Samvashikaran' uses a variety of strategies, although the Atharva Veda mostly employs heightened verbal persuasion.
5. **Ritualistic therapy** (drama and demonstration): drama and demonstration in the form of rituals create a distinct and perplexing technique that can be employed as a supplement to, or in place of, other methods. It is intended for use with illiterates, mad people and children who are unable to comprehend and understand their own mental processes. Typically, it is employed as a supplemental 'sandesh' technique. When teaching a youngster, a teacher must dramatize and illustrate, and the same is true with rituals. The use of symbols in ritualistic healing is accepted by some writers on the Atharva Veda (Karambelkar, 1959). The symbolization and dramatization have a psychological effect, causing the maladaptive behaviour to be cured or changed. This is now known as or is close to *ritualistic therapy* in modern terminology.
6. **'Brahma Kawach'** (psychological defensive belief): The therapies that have been examined thus far have some parallels in Atharva Veda and modern psychotherapies. 'Brahma Kawach', on the other hand, is only found in the Atharva Veda. 'Brahma Kawach' is a form of defence and a psychological term that refers to one's conviction in oneself and support for self-assurance. It instils self-assurance and a belief in one's own ability to defend oneself. 'Brahma Kawach', according to the Atharva Veda, disperses some psychological invisible energy in the surroundings, which functions as a resistance to any destructive energies there.
7. **Utarna** (Transference): It is the process of sending disease symptoms or the disease itself. It is an Atharvenic technique, but its traces can still be found among the Indian indigenous practitioners of today. It has been demonstrated

by Arsh (1999) that it is based on a psychophysiology approach and is not a simple magic or superstition. This technique has been employed in Atharva Veda in two ways: first, to transmit the physical symptoms of disease to plants and animals. In addition, the transference of psychological symptoms to all living beings, including humans, animals, and plants.

8. **Ashwasana and Upchar** (assurance, desensitization, re-education): Ashwasana and upchar are utilized in Atherva Veda as essential preliminary practices and as a supplement to the subsequent therapies for mental disorders. According to Arsh (1999), Ashwasana is assurance, optimism, confidence, and contentment, while upchar is redirecting and re-educating the patient's behaviour. These are prerequisites or necessary conditions for any short-term therapy.
9. **Davaiya havan chikitisa** (spiritual prayer with havan and rituals): Invoking the blessings of various gods and deities, this is a method for the treatment of mental disorders. This is a religious therapy administered by a cleric. Brahma is the name of the cleric who performs the puja and all rituals. In Havan, prayers and offerings are made to the gods, particularly ghee and aromatic herbs are poured into the Agni (fire) as offerings. Priests and patients, and sometimes their relatives, offer prayers.
10. **Tapa/Tyag** (penance/sacrifice): ***Tapa*** is the discipline the ego promises to accept. The physical manifestations of tapa include fasting, standing on one foot, lying prostrate and rolling down a certain distance, enduring extremes of heat and cold, and other methods of inflicting physical agony. The psychological form of tapa may be self-discipline and abstinence, as well as the control of one's impulses, and motivations. While ***Tyag*** implies relinquishing worldly possessions such as valuables, money, etc. In this type of sacrifice or tyag, the ego is relieved of guilt, unburdened, and restored to normalcy. Tyag can be utilized to achieve health, affluence, and prosperity.

6.6 Ayurveda and Psychology

The term 'ayu' refers to all facets of life, from conception to death. Ayurveda denotes the science that explains life as a whole. It is a style of life that outlines what is good or bad for life in terms of diet, medication and conduct. It is predicated on the idea that mental, physical, and spiritual wellness are interdependent and require careful balance. Rather than treating disease, the main goal of Ayurvedic medicine is to promote good health. Treatments, however, could be suggested for particular health issues. When one's mind, body, and spirit are in tune with the cosmos, one will be in good health. A disturbance of this balance might result in illness and bad health. Individual physical and psychological traits come together in the body's constitution, or 'prakruti', which is how the body functions to keep healthy. It is thought that 'prakruti' (human nature) remains constant throughout our lives. However, it can be influenced by how we process food and get rid of junk. Five fundamental components of the universe combine to form each individual: *Earth, space, air, fire, and water*. Three life forces or energies known as 'doshas' are created in the human body when these ingredients unite. They regulate how the body functions. There are three 'doshas': 'Vata' (space and air), 'Pitta' (fire and water), and 'Kapha' (water and earth). Each person receives a special combination of the three 'doshas'. Typically, one 'dosha' is more dominant. Different bodily functions are controlled by each 'dosha'. It is said that the harmony of our 'doshas' affects how likely we are to become ill: physically or mentally.

1. **'Vata Dosha'**: The 'vata dosha' (space and air) is regarded as the most potent of the three. It regulates several fundamental bodily processes, including cell division. It also regulates our blood flow, breathing, mind, heart health, and the capacity to eliminate bodily waste via the intestines. This 'dosha' can be upset by, for example: Consuming dry fruit, fear, grief, eating too soon after a meal and staying up too late. If the 'vata dosha' dominates us, we are more likely to experience: Anxiety, asthma, heart illness, neurological conditions, rheumatoid arthritis and skin issues (Ahuja, 2015).
2. **'Pitta Dosha'**: The digestion, metabolism and several hormones connected to appetite are all under the influence of the 'pitta dosha' (fire and water). Eating sour foods is one thing that can upset this 'dosha' along with consuming hot food, insufficient sleep and too much sun exposure. If the 'pitta dosha' dominates our being, we are more inclined to: Heart disease, Crohn's disease, heartburn that occurs a few hours after eating, high blood pressure, infections and negative feelings which may lead to various mental illnesses.
3. **'Kapha Dosha'**: The 'kapha dosha' (water and earth) regulates the immune system, weight, muscle growth, and body strength and stability. Daytime sleeping, eating even after one's stomach is full, consuming too much salt or water, overindulging in sweets and greed are all things that might cause this 'dosha' to become imbalanced. If the 'kapha dosha' dominates, one is more likely to experience: Cancer, diabetes, post-meal nausea, obesity, asthma and other respiratory conditions (Ahuja, 2015).

Other psychological disorders also are under the influence of the three doshas, which are discussed in later sections.

When talking about Ayurvedic treatment and its psychology; One's individual 'prakruti', dominant 'dosha', and the harmony of all three have a role in how one responds to treatment. Ayurvedic medicine makes it a priority to rid the body of 'ama', or undigested food, which can accumulate inside the body and cause illness, whether physical or mental. 'Panchakarma' is the name of this purification procedure. It is applied to lessen any symptoms and restore equilibrium and harmony. We cannot consider Ayurveda practice without understanding the psychology of 'doshas', 'gunas', and 'karmas'. According to this theory, the body only serves as the location where these imbalances lodge, manifest or lead to illnesses; the mind plays the primary role (Ahuja, 2015). While Ayurveda may appear to be centred on nutritional, herbal and exercise suggestions, it actually involves knowledge of human psychology. Without it, the practitioner is unable to establish the right relationship with the patient to guarantee proper communication and adherence to treatment recommendations. Many acute ailments have been effectively treated by modern medicine, but emotional anguish has increased as a result of several aspects of modern lifestyles that are not in harmony with nature. Psychological illnesses like depression and other mental/psychological disorders are nearly universal in today's society. Even young children frequently have disorders like hyperactivity or attention deficit disorder. An excellent substitute for the modern drug-heavy approach to treating the mind and mental health is nicely outlined in Ayurveda.

6.6.1 Ayurvedic Psychology

Ayurvedic psychology is the study of psychological wellbeing in Ayurveda. All theoretical elements, therapeutic and dietary approaches, and herbal remedies related to enhancing psychological wellbeing within the field of Ayurveda shall be referred to as Ayurvedic psychology (Frawley, 1997; Tirtha, 1998). The three 'doshas' theory offers a framework for Ayurvedic psychology (Rao, 2007). Another subject related to Ayurvedic psychology is Ayurvedic psychiatry. Traditional Ayurvedic psychiatry defined how the 'doshas' and the characteristics of the 'gunas' affected mental disorders. Rhoda (2014) discussed in a study the mark of Aurvedic psychiatry, and Ayurvedic psychological concepts in relation to contemporary diseases and classifications. Due to the mind–body oneness at the core of the discipline, it is vital to define these phrases. The body and mind are fully interconnected and responsible for all physical and mental illnesses, according to the Ayurvedic psychological theory, which emphasizes the necessity of both in achieving perfect health (Lad, 1995). Classical Ayurvedic psychology and psychiatry, or 'bhuta vidya', discussed both endogenous and exogenous sources of illness as well as several varieties of mental illness ('manovikaras') (Fabrega, 2001; Obeyesekere, 1977). The former dealt with imbalances in the psychophysiology brought on by things like the body's constitutional problems, uncontrolled emotions, poor sleep patterns, seasonal changes and genetic susceptibility. Exogenous causes of mental disease linked to paranormal elements include karmic and spiritual tendencies, planetary effects and the deeds of evil paranormal entities (Reddy et al., 1987). Similar to this, research on Ayurvedic effects on mental health is still uncommon. Modern Ayurvedic research has tended to concentrate more on physical aspects of healing. This dearth of study may, in a broader sense, emphasize the mind–body duality in modern scientific research methodologies and priorities (Singh, 2010). The uniqueness of Ayurvedic psychology is built in the understanding that contrasted traits and behaviours promote balance (Frawley, 1997). For instance, a 'vata' person who experiences mental agitation and restlessness is treated with calming activities like oil massage, or calming activities that provide a sense of grounding, like walking in nature, and nourishing dietary options that are gently warming and directly balance the natural lightness and dryness of the 'vata dosha'. Utilizing all five senses is advised by Ayurveda in order to properly address the holistic aspect of treatment (Nichter, 2008). As a result, Ayurveda also includes some of the earliest descriptions of diet, sound healing, massage therapy, aromatherapy and colour therapy (Frawley, 1997; Tirtha, 1998).

The three 'doshas' in 'Sankhya' philosophy also correspond to the three 'gunas', or fundamental mental qualities, known as 'sattva', 'rajas' and 'tamas' (Frawley, 1997). While maintaining a healthy balance of 'rajas' (passion, activity and stimulation) and 'tamas' (dullness, ignorance and dishonesty), Ayurvedic healing modalities are intended to promote 'sattva' (qualities such as purity, honesty and clarity), though from a tactical standpoint, it is occasionally necessary to promote 'rajas' or 'tamas' as a short-term measure when working with a person in a healing process.

The genetic underpinnings of the tridoshic hypothesis are now being examined by a developing area of Ayurvedic study into the biological genome, offering the first attempts in science to support fundamental ideas in Ayurvedic psychology. Through establishing an experimental association between the human leukocyte antigen and the three primary doshic types, Patwardhan et al. (2005) proposed a genetic correlation for the traditional idea of Ayurvedic 'prakruti' (birth constitution). According to the authors, the nuanced interactions between 'vata', 'pitta' and 'kapha' are as unique and personal as a person's DNA. Consequently, the term 'prakruti' has a genetic connotation and may be used as a technique to categorize the human population into large phenotypic clusters.

Ayurvedic psychological research has its evidence in measurement of psycho-Ayurvedic concepts, too. It now includes using doshic theory and other Ayurvedic theoretical components in clinical studies in addition to evaluating them. Suchitra et al. (2010) created a scale to assess the tridoshic symptoms of Ayurvedic Psychosis ('unmaad'). Fifteen Ayurvedic experts, five psychiatrists, and five psychologists were consulted by Suchitra et al. (2010) in order to validate the scale's accuracy and therapeutic applicability. All patients with a diagnosis of schizophrenia unspecified scored above the 75th percentile for the 'pitta' subscale, whereas nearly all patients classified as paranoid schizophrenic did so for the 'vata' subscale. Last but not least, all patients with psychosis not otherwise characterized received 'kapha' subscale scores above the 75th percentile. They found some doshic links to forms of psychosis.

In regard to Ayurvedic psychological (Psycho-Ayurvedic) treatments, the 'shirodhara', a mild therapy for controlling stress and anxiety, is another extensively utilized adjunct therapy to conventional 'panchakarma' therapy. This refers to a technique in which a warm stream of oil is continually applied to the middle of the forehead (or third eye) for 30–45 min in an effort to calm the central nervous system. Traditional practitioners of 'shirodhara' employed it to treat a variety of mental health issues, such as schizophrenia, sleeplessness, anxiety and other affective disorders (Tirtha, 1998). 'Shirodhara' is now widely believed to increase brain coherence between the left and right hemispheres (Tirtha, 1998).

6.6.2 'Tridoshas' ('Vata', 'Pitta' 'Kapha') and Psychology

According to Ayurveda, the physical body of an individual is made up of three basic types termed 'doshas', 'dhatus' and 'malas'. Three 'doshas', seven 'dhatus', and three 'malas' make up the trinity. The 'vata', 'pitta' and 'kapha doshas' ('tridoshas') are the three. The 'trigunas-sattva', 'rajas' and 'tamas' are their psychological counterparts and have an impact on human conduct and how we think and behave. That matter's distinctive property is due to 'una'/characteristics or 'prakruti'. The 'tridoshas' are made up of all five 'mahabhutas', but only one or two of them are more dominant than the others. There can never be a situation when one or both 'mahabhutas' are completely missing. Life cannot exist without all five. For good health, these three 'doshas' must be properly balanced. 'Pitta dosha' is made up of 'tejas' or 'agni' (fire) and 'ap' mahabhutas', whereas 'vata dosha' is made up of 'akasa' (ether) and 'vayu' (air) 'mahabhutas'. The 'ap' (water) and 'prithvi' (earth) 'mahabhutas' make up the 'kapha dosha' (Walia & Singh, 2018).

Due to the correlation between the physical and mental selves, Ayurveda has discussed personality characteristics from both physiological and psychological perspectives. 'Sattva', 'rajas', and 'tamas' are psychological characteristics. The three bodily energies are known as 'vata', 'pitta', and 'kapha' (Mukherjee, 2007).

'Vata Dosha': According to Ayurvedic psychology, people with 'vata' imbalances would show signs of fear, loneliness, excessive anxiety, jitteriness, an extremely restless mind and persistent insomnia. The individual will talk very quickly, jump around in conversation, experience restless legs syndrome and need constant external stimulation. The patient will have an unsteady tongue, rough, brittle nails and very dry skin.

'Pitta Dosha': 'Pitta' imbalances in Ayurvedic psychology cause people to be more prone to anger, criticism, judgement, outbursts and unending analysis. 'Pitta' people demand others to communicate clearly, impatiently and concisely in return. The individual is frequently prematurely greying or going bald, prone to moles and freckles and susceptible to inflammatory diseases.

'Kapha Dosha': According to Ayurvedic psychology, patients with 'kapha' imbalances will display a severe form of despair, avarice, attachment and lethargy. They like routines and are very nurturing and caring. Patients with 'kapha' are often overweight and move and speak slowly. Before responding to a question or expressing an opinion, they might reflect about it for some time. It is challenging to change their thinking after they have made up their mind.

Depending on the relative prominence of the 'doshas' in an individual's body, Charaka and Sushruta identify seven different sorts or groups into which humans might be divided. Ayurveda recognizes 16 different personality types based on the traditional Guna theory in addition to the basic seven varieties of 'prakruti' ('vata', 'pitta', and 'kapha' and their blends). These categories are described in the Charaka and Sushruta Samhitas, respectively. There are 16 different personality types that can be used to categorize all humans, including seven 'sattva' types, six 'rajas' types, and three 'tamas' kinds. 'Brahma', 'Mahendra', 'Varuna', 'Kubera', 'Gandharva', 'Yama', and 'Rishi' are the seven different forms of 'sattva'. 'Asura', 'Rakshasa', 'Paisaca', 'Sarpa', 'Praita', and 'Sakuna' are the six different varieties of 'rajas' type. 'Pasava', 'Matsya', and 'Vanaspatya' are the three varieties of 'tamas' (as per Charaka Samhita and Sushruta Samhita).

The Indian system of medicine, Ayurveda is based on the two principles: (1) 'Panchamahabhuta', which describes the five elements that make up the physical cosmos, including the human body (macrocosm and microcosm), and (2) the foundation of every person's constitution is the 'tridoshas', which are the three 'doshas' of 'vata', 'pitta', and 'kapha'. An individual's personality is referred to as their 'prakruti', which is a Sanskrit word that signifies their nature or natural form of constitution, in the Indian medical system of Ayurveda. It speaks of one's own constitution, which is unique to each person and is governed by their own physiology (Ravi et al., 2013). The three 'doshas', control all bodily processes on the physical, mental and emotional levels. As a result, an individual's 'prakruti' consists of their physiological, psychological and behavioural characteristics.

6.6.3 Concept of 'Prakruti' (Nature/Character/Personality)

Every person has a distinct fingerprint, just as every human being upon conception has a different balance of the three 'doshas'. This creates 'prakruti', which establishes a person's identity and is based on a specific ratio of the 'tridoshas' whichcontrols a person's physiological, psychological and physical traits. The neurological and musculoskeletal systems are governed by 'vata dosha' (Menon, 2016). The psychosomatic makeup known as 'prakruti' is composed of the triads, which have fixed proportions in our bodies at the time of conception. Understanding the origin, classification and features of 'prakruti' in Ayurveda, further aids in comprehending the physiological, psychological and behavioural facets of an individual. The Sanskrit 'sloka' in Charak Samhita-Indriya Sthanam *1/5*, describes postnatal elements that affect how one's 'prakruti', or personality, develops (Prasuna et al., 2014). Charak describes:

1. **'Jati Prasaktha'**: This is the personality of the human race or religion into which a person isborn.
2. **'Kula Prasaktha'**: This is the birth family/effect.
3. **'Desha Anupatini'**: These are one's habitat's characteristics.
4. **'Kala Anupatini'**: This is a season or period.
5. **'Vayas Anupatini'**: These are life stages.
6. **'Prati Atmaniyata'**: This is founded on primal instincts.

Therefore, 'jati' and 'kula'; families with distinct lifestyles, eating habits, cultures, belief systems, and thinking patterns; along with 'desha' (location or geographic location), 'kala' (season), 'vayas' (age) and 'pratiatmaniyata' (the distinct instincts) form the basis of each person's unique physical, mental and verbal characteristics. Thus,

Ayurveda provides a thorough and detailed explanation of the variables affecting a person's fundamental build. The idea of the 'Tridoshas' offers a framework for Ayurvedic psychology. In relation to the 'doshas', the aetiology of physical and mental disorders, along with related therapeutic interventions and dietary changes, are proposed. Ayurvedic psychology could be especially relevant to the developing subject of transpersonal psychology and could gain from transpersonal research techniques that respect the Ayurvedic system's holistic approach (Daniel, 2014).

Based on the 'Tridoshas', 'prakruti' is divided into 'Dosha Prakruti' and 'Deha Prakruti'. There are seven of them: three 'Ekadoshaja', each of which has one dominant 'dosha'; three 'Dvi' (two) doshaja', each of which has two dominant 'doshas'; and one 'Sama prakruti', or 'Sama doshaja', which has three 'doshas' in a balanced state. 'Prakruti' offers a manual for healthy living that is individually tailored to each person's lifestyle (Singer & Le Vine, 2001). Classical literature describe 'Pancha bhuta Prakruti', which is based on the supremacy of the five elements: 'Prithvi', 'Ap', 'Tejas', 'Vayu' and 'Aakasha', as having three forms of 'Manasa Prakruti' based on the 'trigunas': 'Sattva', 'Rajas', and 'Tamas' (As per, Sushrutha Samhitha and Ashtanga Hrydaya). Based on the dominant 'dosha' at the time of conception, an individual's 'prakruti' might be compared to their psychophysiological composition (Prasuna et al., 2014), as shown below:

'Vata Prakruti': They lack confidence in their courage, memory, thinking and friendship; they are unable to regulate their senses; they attach and detach quickly; they are not civilized; they are unpleasant and restless. They have an impetuous personality, are quick to pick up new information but forget it quickly, are easily alarmed, jealous, unlucky and wrathful.

'Pitta Prakruti': They are proud, courageous, and gifted with good intelligence. They are fiercely competitive and envious, fear discomfort, yearn for grandeur, and like compliments. They behave well, are tidy, kind to their dependents and exhibit cultured behaviour.

'Kapha Prakruti': They are obedient to teachers, have solid intelligence, and are righteous and benevolent in character. They also refrain from using harsh or abusive language. They frequently take their timc and are sluggish while learning new things, but once they master a task, they have good recall and retention. They are well-educated, respectable, extraordinarily charitable, forgiving by nature, civilized and have solid scriptural knowledge and opinions.

Literature on Ayurveda also discusses 'Manasa Prakruti', which is based on 'Trigunas' and 'Sankhya' philosophy. Based on the 'Trigunas', there are three forms of 'Manasa Prakruti': 'Sattvika', 'Rajasika', and 'Tamasika'. The three 'gunas': 'amas', 'Rajas', and 'Sattva' are the three crucial elements of thought, just like 'Deha' or 'Dosha Prakruti'. 'Sattva' stands for perfect morality and wisdom. 'Rajas' stands for rage, arrogance and jealousy. 'Tamas' is a representation of apathy, ignorance and confusion. 'Rajas' and 'Tamas' are categorized as 'Manodoshas', whilst 'Tridoshas' are known as 'Saririkadoshas' (as per Vaghbhatta, Ashtanga Hrydaya; Sarira Sthanam, 3/83).

The triads are biological embodiments of the body that are in charge of both pathological illnesses and physiological processes that are in a state of homeostasis. Movement and dynamism require 'vata'. 'Vata dosha' that is vitiated is the cause of a large number of nerve and mental disorders. 'Vataja' is primarily associated with fear, anxiety, hallucinations, delusions and psychosis. 'Pitta' governs the psychological aspects of intelligence, reasoning, discriminating and judgement, or what is known as the mind's illuminating capacity. Aggression, intolerance, antisocial behaviour, impatience and angry outbursts are all symptoms of vitiated 'Pitta dosha' (Venkobarao, 2002). On a psychological level, 'kapha' controls feelings and the mind's ability to cling onto forms. Although the mind becomes more stable and at peace as a result, there may be a delay in mental development. 'Kapha' personalities are characterized by passivity, apathy, withdrawal, melancholy and depression (Daniel, 2014; Venkobarao, 2002).

'Tridoshas' leave behind psychological imprints known as 'Trigunas' (Shilpa & Murthy, 2011). The seven-fold categorization of humans according to their 'gunas' is comparable to their seven-fold categorization according to their 'dosha prakruti'. This shows that a person's physical makeup determines whether they have the related psychological traits or not, as the two are linked. The core of Ayurvedic knowledge is the interaction between the intellect ('sattva'), soul ('atman') and body ('sarira') in a tripod analogy.

6.6.4 Maharishi Charaka

Eight crucial psychological components that are adversely impacted in diverse ways in all psychiatric diseases are described by Charaka in his book (*Charaka Samhita).* These factors: 'manas' (mind), 'buddhi' (intellect), 'smriti' (memory), 'srijna jnana' (orientation and responsiveness), 'bhakti' (devotion), 'shila' (habits), 'cheshta' (psychomotor activity), and 'achara' (conduct) have an impact on the psychopathological condition. Charaka Samhita places more stress on the idea that existence is a self-aware field of pure consciousness and natural intelligence, where the knower and the known are one, than other important Ayurvedic works like Sushruta Samhita and Ashtanga Hrdayam (Walia & Singh, 2018).

The three varieties of the mind-psyche as described in various ways earlier; are 'sattvika' (pure), 'rajasika', and 'tamasika'. In contrast to 'rajasika' and 'tamasika', who may be seen as partially flawed due to the presence of characteristics such as agitation and ignorance in them, respectively, the pure is stated to be without faults due to possessing some good factor. Each one of these three sorts of psyche has many subcategories of relative degrees and variances in how mind and body interact, depending on the species. Psyche follows the body and vice versa. In the context of personality profiles, seven different 'Sattvika' types, six different 'Rajasika' types, and three different 'Tamasika' types are found in Charaka's writings (Mukherjee, 2007). There are countless variations among the three sorts of mental faculties. The seven varieties of the 'Sattvika' mental faculty are determined by the temperaments of 'Brahma', 'Arsa', 'Aindra', 'Yamya', 'Varuna', 'Kaubera' and 'Gandharava'. Further, 'Asura', 'Raksasa', 'Pisaca', 'Sarpa', 'Preta' and 'Sakuni' dispositions are six different varieties of 'Rajasa' mental faculties. The 'Pasu' (beast), 'Matsya' (fish), and 'Vanaspati' (vegetable life) dispositions determine which of the three varieties of 'Tamasa' mental faculties exist (Mukherjee, 2007). The seven 'Sattvika' types of mental faculty are:

1. **Brahma**: Purity, love of truth and self-control; discernment; material and spiritual knowledge; power of exposition, reply and memory; freedom from fervour, anger, greed and ego; ignorance; jealousy; dejection; intolerance; and a disposition that is equally favourable to all creatures are all characteristics shared by 'Brahma' (Sharma, 1981). Such a person should be referred to as a Brahma type (similar to Brahma) in Ayurvedic psychology because they are pure, true to their word, in control of themselves, distribute shares, endowed with learning, understanding, speaking and contradicting; and with memory. They are also free of passion, anger, greed, conceit, confusion, envy, exhilaration and intolerance.
2. **Arsa (Rsis)**: Dedication to religious practices, study, sacred vows, oblations and celibacy; a friendly demeanour; freedom from arrogance, ego, attachment, hatred, ignorance, greed and rage; intellectual prowess and eloquence; and the capacity for understanding and memory (Sharma, 1981). A person who practices sacrifices, study, vows, oblations and celibacy; who is devoted to guests, has conquered pride, conceit, attachment, aversion, confusion, greed and anger; and who is endowed with the powers of imagination, speaking, understanding and retention should be referred to as 'Arsa' (similar to sages) in the mind.
3. **Aindra (Indra)**: Lord-like authority, the ability to execute sacred ceremonies, bravery, strength and beauty, the absence of malice, foresight and a commitment to doing good deeds in order to gain money and satisfy one's wants in the right way are all qualities that one must possess (Sharma, 1981). One who is in charge and whose words are pleasing, who makes sacrifices, who acts bravely, vigorously, soothingly, and is unhindered, who is foresighted, who is committed to virtue, wealth and pleasure Such a person ought to be referred to as 'Aindra' (similar to Indra) in psyche (Sharma & Dash, 1977). They are independent and assertive.
4. **Yamya (Yama)**: Respect for the appropriateness of action, timing, nonviolence, readiness to act, remembrance and lordship, as well as freedom from attachment, enmity, hatred and ignorance (Sharma, 1981). Such a person should be referred to as 'Yamya' (similar to Yama, God of Death) in the mind for keeping records of their behaviour, acting at the right time, being unbeatable, endowed with promptness and memory, achieving dominance, free from attachment, envy, dislike and bewilderment. These people are forceful.
5. **Varuna (similar to Varuna, Water God)**: Bravery, patience, purity, and dislike of impurity; observance of religious rites; love of aquatic activities; dislike of mean-spirited behaviour; and appropriate expression of wrath and pleasure (Sharma, 1981). Such a person should be referred to as 'Varuna' in the mind

since they are brave, persistent, clean, dislike uncleanliness, involved in sacrifice, enjoy water-related activities (swimming, etc.), and have unhindered actions. These people are calm, collected and traditional.

6. **Kaubera (similar to Kubera, God of Wealth)**: Possession of station, honour, luxuries and attendants; consistent preference for righteous deeds, money and the gratification of wishes; purity; and preference for recreational pleasures (Sharma, 1981). Such a person should be referred to as 'Kaubera' in the mind because of their status, conceit, enjoyment and retinue; constant engagement in virtue, money and pleasure; clean, easy movements; and manifesting of rage and favour. These people are confident and at ease.
7. **Gandharava (similar to Gandharva, Celestial Nymph)**: Expertise in poetry, stories, historical accounts and epics; a lifelong love of smells, garlands, colognes, women's clothing, and passion (Sharma, 1981); a penchant for dancing, singing, music, and praise. In terms of their psyche (Sharma & Dash, 1977), this kind of person is referred to as 'Gandharava' These people are quick, carefree, optimistic and gregarious. Only in this 'Sattvika' kind is the preference for the company of ladies indicated. So, this kind of 'Sattvika' may occasionally be jovial and outgoing (Sharma, 1981).

As a result, due to their positive character, the pure psyche (also known as 'Sattvika', individuals of pure and good disposition), has been split into seven categories. Due to the prevalence of the aforementioned character, 'Brahma' is regarded as the purest being (Sharma & Dash, 1977).

There are six varieties of the 'Rajasika' type of mental faculty, which denotes a wrathful disposition:

1. **'Asura' (Villain)**: Traits include: Bravado, malice, enmity, dominion, disguising one's identity, intimidating appearance, ruthlessness, and self-praise (Sharma, 1981). 'Asure' (similar to 'Asura') should be thought of as being brave, violent, backbiting, supreme, dishonest, furious, ruthless and self-praising. These people are tenacious, cunning and outspoken.
2. **'Raksasa' (Demonic Disposition)**: Traits include: Intemperance, unrelenting rage, cruelty, a gluttonous appetite for meat and other non-vegetarian foods, an excessive amount of sleep and laziness and an envious nature (Sharma, 1981). A person should be viewed as 'Raksasa' (similar to Raksasa) in psychology if they are intolerant, persistently angry, cruel, enjoy overeating, have a strong craving for meat, indulge in sleep and physical activity and are envious. In short, Raksasa type people like non-vegetarian food very much (Sharma & Dash, 1977).
3. **Paisacha (Malevolent Being of Devilish Character)**: Exhibit the following traits: gluttony, a penchant for staying with women in lonely places, a dislike of hygiene, cowardice, a scary demeanour and the adoption of strange diets and routines (Sharma, 1981). Also, if they are gluttonous, fond of women, wanting to meet women in private, dirty, disliking the clean, frightened, terrifying and regularly engaging in improper diet and behaviour, such a person should be taken as 'Paisaca' (similar to 'Psaca') in Ayurvedic psychology (Sharma & Dash, 1977). Such individuals have more sexual orientation to opposite sex and men feel much

attracted to women. The first time that attraction to women was described was in the 'Gandharba' kind of 'Sattvika', but the level of desire for women in the 'Paisaca' type of 'Rajasika' is more unacceptable.

4. **Sarpa (Snake)**: Traits include: Sharp reactions, excessive indolence, strolling, consuming meals, and turning to other routines when feeling terrified, which are all examples of cowardice. They are also examples of bravery when having a wrathful temperament (Sharma, 1981). Such a person should be regarded as 'Sarpa' (similar to Sarpa or serpent) in the mind since they are robust while angry, but afraid otherwise. They are sharp, active, and intimidate others wherever they go. This personality is tense rather than gluttonous.
5. **Praita (Dead or Departed Spirit)**: These personalities show excessive desire for food, excessively painful character traits and past behaviours, envy and carry out actions without discrimination, and with excessive greediness or inaction. Such a person should be regarded as 'Praita' type.
6. **Sakuna (Sakuni or Bird)**: Traits include: Passionate attachment, excessive eating and exercise, shakiness, harshness and refusal to give in (Sharma, 1981). Such a person should be regarded as 'Sakuna' (similar to 'sakuni' or birds) in psychology if they are passionate, continuously indulge in food and hobbies, unstable, intolerable and lack hoarding tendencies (Sharma & Dash, 1977). These people lack discipline, are dependent on groups, uptight and happy-go-lucky.

The three varieties of the 'Tamasika' type of mental faculty, which denotes ignorance, are:

1. **Pasava (Animal)**: Those people showing traits like repudiating, lacking intelligence, having a dislike for food and behaviour, indulging in sexual activity and sleeping excessively should be taken as 'Pasava' (similar to 'pasu' or animals) (Sharma & Dash, 1977). Such people are undisciplined, less intelligent and outgoing.
2. **Matsya (Fish)**: Cowardice, lack of intelligence, a voracious appetite, instability, an unrelenting drive for anger, a preference for constant movement and a longing for water (Sharma, 1981) are the main characteristics of 'Matsya' kind of people. A person should be viewed as 'Matsya' (similar to fish) if they are timid, foolish, gluttonous, unstable, continuously gripped by passion and rage, always on the move and fond of water (Sharma & Dash, 1977). These people lack discipline, are less bright, are reliant on groups and are uptight.
3. **Vanaspatya (Vegetable Life)**: Those with traits like gastronomic overindulgence, intellectual underdevelopment and indolence (Sharma, 1981) should be regarded as 'Vanaspatya' (akin to the 'Vanaspati' plant). Such people lack intelligence and depend on their group. This personality type resembles the idiot personality type (Chandra, 1978).

6.6.5 *Maharishi Shushruta*

Mukherjee (2007) discussed Shushruta's thoughts on personality types.

First, '**Sattvika**' **features**. Those who fit into one of these seven categories are said to have a 'Sattvika' mental temperament (Visagratna, 1981): (1) features of a '**Brahma-Kaya**' person include cleanliness of person and behaviour, faith in God, regular Vedic reading, veneration for elders and preceptors, hospitality to others and performance of religious rites; (2) a '**Mahendra-Kaya**' person possesses the following qualities: bravery, leadership, frequent discussion of the Astras, care for servants and dependents and magnanimity of spirit; (3) a '**Varuna-Kaya**' individual has a preference for exposure to cold, is patient, has brown eyes, has golden hair and has a beautiful voice; (4) the characteristics of a '**Kauvera-Kaya**' individual are the ability to arbitrate conflicts, endure hardships, acquire and accumulate riches and have children or be fertile; (5) a '**Gandharva-Kaya**' individual has the following characteristics: they enjoy wearing garlands and perfumes, singing and listening to music and making love; (6) **Yamya-Kaya** people have a strong sense of duty, are prompt, firm in their actions, brave, have good memories, are pure, and lack wrath, illusion, fear and malice; and (7) the characteristics of a **Rsi-Kaya** person are divine contemplation, vow observance, total celibacy, 'Homas' (sacrificial fire), celebration of religious sacrifices, knowledge, wisdom and cultivation of divine or spiritual science.

Second, '**Rajasika**' **features**. The following are six 'Rajasika' mentality types (Visagratna, 1981): (1) people who fit the '**Asura**' **type** tend to be wealthy, terrible, valiant, irascible, envious of other men's success, gluttons, and fond of eating by themselves without sharing with anybody else; (2) a person of the '**Sarpa**' **type** is hurried while eating and having sexual relations, laborious, cowardly, angry and irritated; (3) a person of the '**Akuna**' **type** is gluttonous, immature in sexual issues, agitated and fickle; (4) '**Raksasa**' **type** individuals are isolated in their behaviour, furious, envious of others' success, outwardly pious, incredibly conceited and uninformed; (5) the traits of a '**Paisacha**' **type** of person include consuming food that has been consumed by another person, having a quick temper, acting rashly, being shameless and coveting the things of wome; (6) **Preta-type** people are completely ignorant of their obligations, lazy, miserable, envious, covetous and niggardly.

Third, the three '**Tamasika**' personality types: (1) the characteristics of a '**Pasava**' **type** of person are perverse intelligence, austerity, frequent sexual dreams and an inability to perceive or ascertain anything; (2) the characteristics of the '**Matsya**' **kind** of person are unsteadiness, ignorance, fear, a preference for intermissive argument and oppression and a yearning for water; and (3) the traits of a '**Vanaspati**' **type** of individual include a preference for remaining put, continual eating, and a lack of sincerity, piety, wealth and pleasure (Visagratna, 1981).

'Prakruti' (Temperaments): Mukherjee (2007) further discussed the concept of temperament discussed in Shushruta's Samhita. Due to the disordered 'doshas' of the body's involvement, which can occur singly, in combination with another 'dosha', or in all three at once, there are seven possible sorts of temperaments ('prakruti') for individuals. The predominance of a specific 'dosha' during a person's generation determines their temperament ('prakruti'), which is distinguished by that 'dosha' (Visagratna, 1981).

'Vataja' temperament: A person with the temperament of 'Vata' is awake, averse to bathing and cold contact, ungainly, thievish, vain, dishonest and fond of music; the soles of the feet and the palms of the hands are much fissured; the individual frequently plays rough sports and has grisly facial hair, fingernails and hair; the person is also hot-tempered and prone to biting their fingernails and grinding their teeth (when asleep). These people's bodies are marked by a great number of conspicuous veins ('Dhamani'), and morally, they are impetuous, shaky in their friendship, ungrateful, lean and rough. They also have inconsistent habits and a fickle disposition. They move quickly on foot and dream in their sleep of conquering the skies. Their eyes never stop moving. Their thoughts are never stable. They are unable to amass much wealth, make few friends and speak incoherently (Visagratna, 1981).

'Pittvaja' temperament: 'Pittvaja' temperament people sweat profusely and smell like the field. Their limbs have an amorphous form and a yellowish colour. Such a person has copper-coloured fingernails, eyes, lips, palate, tongue, soles and palms. With wrinkles, baldness, and grey hair, they have an unattractive appearance. These people also eat a lot, dislike heat, and have a short fuse when angry. They have average strength and make it to middle age. They love to dominate the conversation and are intelligent with a strong recall. They defend the suppliant and are frequently linked to suppuration in the oral cavity (Visagratna, 1981). They are never overcome by fear and never yield to a strong adversary.

'Kaphaja' temperament: The people with this temperament would be strong, grateful, self-controlled, forgiving, unselfish and have a serene aspect. They do not form opinions prematurely and are quick to express hostility. Their curling, raven-black hair is black, and they have white eyes. They enjoy success in life. Their voice has a lion's roar, a rain cloud's rumblings, or a Mrudanga's tone to it. In their sleep, they have visions of sizeable lakes or pools that are decorated with countless full-bloom lotus flowers, swans and 'Cakravakas'. Their limbs are proportionately and symmetrically grown, with cool effulgence radiating from them. Their eyes are slightly reddish in the corners. They possess traits that bear the 'Sattvika' imprint, including the ability to endure discomfort and exhaustion, and respect for their superiors. They have faith in the astras, are unwavering in their friendship, experience no vagaries of fortune, make significant presents after careful consideration, are reliable and consistently obey their preceptors (Visagratna, 1981).

A person's temperament never changes; it doesn't get worse or weaker. In any specific situation, a change, reduction, or deterioration should be seen as a sign that someone is near to death (Mukherjee, 2007). Even if it offends others, a person's temperament is of no hardship to him or her. The 'Vata prakruti', the 'Taijasa prakruti', and the 'pya (watery) prakruti', which have characteristics that, respectively, correspond to the three temperaments mentioned earlier—air, fire, and water—have been classified as the temperaments of people who believe that their temperaments originate in the physical elements of the body. A person with the '**Parthiva**' **temperament** is tall and has firm, powerful and muscular limbs. The '**Nabhasa**' **temperament** is characterized by piety, longevity and huge aural cavities. The qualities of the different mental temperaments are used to categorize them (Visagratna, 1981).

There are no known references to animal psychology research in Ayurveda (Sengupta and Sengupta, 1916). 'Slesma' or 'kapha' aids the body by steadiness, smoothness, by serving the units, and so forth, while 'pitta' (bile) aids the body by digestive function, heat, function of sight imagination ('medha'), power of understanding ('dhi'), courage ('saurya') and softness of the body. 'Vata', 'pitta' and 'kapha' thereby carry out both bodily and mental functions. 'Kapha prakruti', or the predominance of 'Sattva guna', is described by Sushruta as 'Sattva pradhana'. The 'Kaphaja' and 'Sattvika' types are recognized in Sushruta Samhita, but 'Vataja' and 'Pittvaja' temperaments are not specifically stated. 'Pittvaja' temperament is described as a synthesis of 'Raja guna' and 'Sattva guna' (Visagratna, 1981). The 'Vataja' temperament can coexist with 'Tama' and 'Raja guna'. 'Rajas' and 'Tamas' are 'doshas' of the mind, while 'sattva' is a characteristic of the mind (Dasgupta, 1952).

6.6.6 Psychology in Ayurveda

Ayurveda does a good job of describing psychology. The three components, Ayurveda, yoga, and Adhyatma are life's tripod. The subject of the mind is at the heart of the entire yoga science. Through the fundamental requirement of 'Aarogya', Ayurveda seeks to achieve 'moksha'. To acquire 'moksha' through yoga and Adhyatma, the primary subject of yoga science is 'ma-nasvyadhi' (mental disorders). Shukla and Tripathi (2011) suggest Ayurvedic explanations for the causes of 'manasarogas' (psychological disorders). This aphorism suggests a much more enigmatic meaning, a combination or contact of sensory organs with the three different categories of objects. The natural and pure manner is beneficial and healthy. Little or no contact and excessive or unwholesome contact ('atiyoga') cause harm to the organ in question and cause pain. The term 'mind' in Ayurveda refers to the linked internal organ. Internal organs are also affected when an exterior organ is destroyed. This results in the illness 'manasa'. Intellectual derailment is referred to as 'pragyaa-paradha'. This amounts to intellectual heresy. When someone is aware of the negative effects of their behaviour but still chooses to carryon, they are acting against their intelligence. This propensity is present at every stage of life. The intellectual blasphemy components are allures, lust and passionate cravings. Krishna in the Bhagvad Gita says: '*Chanchalam hi manaha*' (mind is unstable): the original character of the mind is one of changeability, instability, and impulsivity. Like a butterfly, the mind flits quickly back and forth. Thousands of crimes are committed every day throughout the world as a result of intellectual blasphemy, as we can see. Due to a lack of control over the mind and sensory organs, the current state of the globe is fast deteriorating.

6.6.6.1 The Mind in Ayurveda

'जैसा खाये अन्न, वैसा बने मन।'

The mind becomes like the food one eats.

Indian Proverb

This proverb emphasizes the importance of the food we consume in forming a healthy mind. Ayurveda also describes how the micro part of the food becomes the mind in our body. As described in Indian philosophy, food is the 'Brahmn' ('अन्नं ब्रह्म').

The physiology and pathology of the physical body are influenced by the mind. The creators of Ayurveda were aware of this reality. As a result, Ayurveda is described as a life philosophy and science. One of the six main philosophical schools of ancient India, Sankhya philosophy, or 'shad dharshana', is where the Ayurvedic understanding of the mind originates. According to Sankhya, the four strata of the mind are as follows (Frawley, 2012): (1) 'Chitta' (conditioned consciousness); (2) 'Buddhi' (wise decision-making); (3) 'Mana's (mind, creative ability); and (4) 'Ahamkara' (Ego). According to Charaka, the first two humours are imbalances, whereas the third humour represents the natural state of an unperturbed mind. Additionally, it is believed that the mind functions as a conduit for consciousness, or 'srotas'. It starts in the physical heart, travels through the body, and terminates in the five sense organs (eyes, ears, nose, tongue and skin) (Lad, 2002).

If we have a look at the anatomy and physiology of the mind in Ayurveda, we find that numerous routes exist in the Ayurvedic tradition to transport nutrition and energy. These channel systems proceed from a *root* to a *passageway* and then to an *opening*, and they have both corporeal and noncorporeal characteristics (Lad, 2002). The root of the intellect lies in the heart, and the ten vessels, which are partially correlated with the sense organs, are: (1) two nostrils, (2) two ears, (3) two eyes, (4) mouth, (5) rectum and (6) urethra. These passages move throughout the entire body (Welch, 2005). 'Sushumna', the tenth vessel, is rooted in the heart and emerges from the crown of the head (Welch, 2005). Since the body contains mental pathways, there is reciprocal connection between the body and the mind (Dash, 2008; Welch, 2005). As a result, a physical imbalance may affect the mind, and a vitiated mind may result in physical disruption (Welch, 2005). The relationship between the body, the intellect, the soul and the senses is explained in classic Ayurvedic writings (Dash, 2008). The interaction of the sensory faculties with their perceived objects affects the mental state. The intellect looks for sensory stimulation in concert with the work of the soul. Vitiation of the mind is prone to happen if the sensory input is overwhelming, inadequate or incorrect.

Development of a Healthy Mind: The healthy development of the personality and the uninterrupted flow of 'prana' are nourished by adequate mental digestion of internally and externally originating stimuli. When a person's mind is operating normally and free of illness, evidence of good mental digestion are visible. Svoboda (1999) listed six indicators of a healthy mental diet, stating that the following conditions must be met: (1) there is no mental discomfort following the ingestion of the desired quantity of sense objects; (2) the mind does not feel jaded and full afterwards; (3) no unfavourable emotions are produced while one is processing new information; (4) one can recall one's experiences from memory with ease and accuracy and can communicate them; (5) one's sleep following indulging is sound and enjoyable, without unsettling dreams (which are an indication of 'ama' or undigested experiences); and (6) after an adequate amount of time, the need for additional sensory gratification appears.

In discussing Ayurvedic ways to develop a healthy mind, the process is described as cultivating 'sattva' ('sattavajaya'). Ayurvedic psychology aims to alter the mind's energetics (Halpern, 2010). Making the 'rajas' (the sharp mind) tranquil and the 'tamas' (the dull mind) sharp ('sattva'). According to the Charaka Samhita, one should treat the mind with knowledge, specific knowledge, restraint, memory and concentration (Van Loon, 2002), and the person with a strong mind who does not indulge in meat or wine; who eats only healthy food; and who remains clean both physically and mentally does not become affected by 'unmaad' (insanity) (Ashtanga Hrdayam, Chap. 5. Treatment of Insanity/Verse-59). The process of regaining mental health involves developing the clarity of mind that Ayurveda refers to as 'sattva'. This type of therapy has historically been the principal way for treating mental illness and is one of the three basic treatment modalities (Behere, 2013; Frawley & Halpern, 2006). Frawley outlines the three phases of mental recovery in his book as follows (Frawley, 1997): (1) Creating 'Rajas' or Breaking 'Tamas': Changing mental stagnation into self-driven action; (2) Calming 'Rajas' or Building 'Sattva': Changing from self-serving behaviour to altruistic behaviour; and (3) 'Sattva' Perfection: The transition from meditation to selfless service.

Finding the dominating 'guna' in the mind is crucial to establish the beginning point. To break up the stasis if the mind is tamasic, rajasic, or energetic, therapies are required before switching to sattvic, or calming, therapies. Halpern (2010) describes how to cultivate 'sattva': (1) Spend more time outdoors to help the tranquil and harmonious impressions to permeate consciousness through all of the five senses; (2) Practise meditation to calm the mind and increase self-awareness; (3) Use all eight limbs of yoga help to build 'sattva' by establishing a set of guidelines for both internal and exterior behaviour; (4) Refrain from letting the media affect the individual: TV is rajasic and disrupts the mind; and (5) Follow a sattvic diet, which consists of fresh, organic and pure vegetarian food. Further, Halpern claims that maintaining regular daily practices ('dinacharya') is crucial to the treatment of mental disease (Frawley & Halpern, 2006). Establishing wholesome practices strengthens mental fortitude, or 'ojas', and balances the mobile effects of 'vata dosha' inside the mind. A clear and tranquil mind can be developed by leading a healthy lifestyle. Circadian medicine, which is still in its infancy, is the study of how bodies and minds function according to a 24-h cycle. Incongruent circadian rhythms have been related in studies to depression, bipolar disorder, and schizophrenia (Karatsoreos, 2014).

6.6.6.2 Ayurvedic Signs of Mental Health

Each person has a distinct personality, or 'manasprakruti', which the three 'gunas' and the five components of Ayurveda use to characterize (Halpern, 2010). The three body humours; 'vata', 'pitta', and 'kapha', as well as the two mental traits ('gunas'); rajas or tamas, traditionally contribute to mental imbalances or 'manasvikruti' (Halpern, 2010). Through the eight-fold examination procedure, ayurvedic doctors ('vaidyas') or practitioners can ascertain a patient's current psychological state ('manas vikruti'), which is called 'ashta vidya pariksha'. Walia and Singh (2018) identify Ayurvedic signs of mental health as: (1) Having a good memory; (2) Eating the correct things at the proper times; (3) Being aware of one's obligations; (4) Being aware of oneself and beyond oneself; (5) Keeping oneself clean and hygienic; (6) Being enthusiastic in what one does; (7) Being shrewd and discriminating; (8) Being bold; (9) Showing persistence; (10) Remaining upbeat no matter what the circumstances; (11) Showing positivity in the face of challenges; (12) Having exceptional mental acuity; (13) Showing self-reliance; (14) Following a moral code and (15) Having the capacity to move forward unwaveringly in the face of adversity.

The mind controls the body, and the body controls the complete physiology after that; as a result, one with a pure mind has divine strength, extra-perceptory powers and other abilities. This is similar to how the body follows the mind when both 'rajas' and 'tamas doshas' are present. As a result, people are greatly influenced by their mentality. There are several types of mental faculties as well, such as the satvikamental faculty, the rajasmental faculty and the tamasmental faculty, much as physiologically atominated constitutions are extensively examined in Ayurveda. Due to their close connection, the mind and body interact with one another. One must suffer when the other is ill. Other mental illnesses include 'unmaad' (insanity and its numerous varieties), 'apasmar' (epilepsy and its various types), and others. The other general disorders may also appear when rajas & tamas imbalance occur, which are 'lobha' (greed), 'krodha' (anger) and 'dvesha' (malice). Kumar and Chaudhari (2016) note the following common characteristics to help identification: Eyes contracting and blinking excessively; runny nose and excessive salivation; lack of or overwhelming inclination towards food; frequent complaints of giddiness; weird words and conduct; unsteadiness in the fingers and feet; unnecessary timidity at times and uncalled-for rage over trifles.

There are numerous illnesses that are directly related to 'pragyaaparadha' (Shukla and Tripathi, 2011). Exogenous illnesses brought on by bad spirits, poison, wind, fire and external assaults are all primarily the results of mental capacity deficiencies. Lamentation, dread, rage, misery, self-conceit, hatred and disdain are all considered to be mental illnesses. It is believed that 'trishna' (desire) is the true and root cause of all illnesses. 'Trishna' can be translated as a strong desire for something. When someone longs for something and doesn't receive it or doesn't get it to their satisfaction, frustration, tension and, ultimately, mental illness result. One is therefore advised to stay away from desires and longings. Such a habit can help prevent countless diseases and support good health maintenance.

The Origin of Mental Illness: According to Halpern, all mental illnesses begin with a lack of clarity ('sattva') in the mind (Halpern, 2010). This illustrates the central theme of Ayurveda as a whole, namely that individuals lose their actual essence as spirit when they are born. Ayurveda traditionally identifies the following three disease-causing factors (Halpern, 2010): (1) Intellectual crime ('pragyaparadha'), (2) Misusing the senses ('asatmendriyartha samyoga') and (3) Time-zand motion-related decay ('parinama'). These reasons highlight how closely connected body, mind and spirit are in Ayurveda. The first two factors are crucial to understanding how mental illness begins. Making poor decisions, like staying up too late or indulging in comfort food that is harmful, is considered to be intellectual crime. Injury to oneself or others, such as cutting, anorexia nervosa, or physical abuse, would be considered a sign of serious mental illness. Charaka categorizes the second cause, improper use of the senses, into three categories: inadequate use, excessive use and improper use. The mind and sense organs are closely connected. The rising use of touchscreen devices and exposure to the media is one of today's most significant challenges. At the very least, these gadgets take our attention away from the outside world; at the worst, excessive smartphone use has been linked to depressive symptoms like insomnia and increased stress (Sara et al., 2011). An imbalance of 'tridoshas' and 'gunas' is intended to be corrected through the yogic technique of 'pratyahar', or the withdrawal of the sense inwards. Physical imbalances resulting from the three pillars of health may also contribute to mental disorders. The primary importance of nutrition, sleep and the control of sexual energy, or 'brahamacharya', is acknowledged by Ayurveda. The mind can become out of balance when the physical humours, or 'doshas', are out of equilibrium. More fear, concern and anxiety will be displayed in 'vata' mental imbalances. 'Pitta' out of equilibrium will display as rage, violence and anger, while lethargy and apathy are the symptoms of a 'kapha' mental imbalance (Halpern, 2010).

6.6.6.3 Classification of Mental Illness

The Charaka Samhita only recognizes one type of mental illness: insanity or 'unmaad', in contrast to the contemporary Diagnostic and Statistical Manual of Mental Disorders, which recognizes hundreds of diagnosable psychological disorders. 'Unmaad' is described in traditional texts as excessive wondering of the brain, mind and memory (Van Loon, 2002). This is triggered by eating unclean food, blasphemy and mental shock (Van Loon, 2002). The irritated 'doshas' enter the mental channels from the 'hrudaya', the emotional centre and seat of intelligence, where the root of 'unmaad' begins, leading to an imbalance in the mind (Van Loon, 2002). Charaka Samhita gives the traditional divisions of 'unmaad' as: 'Vataja', caused by vitiation by the 'vata dosha'; 'Pittaja', caused by vitiation by the 'pitta dosha'; 'Kaphaja', caused by vitiation by the 'kapha dosha' and 'Sannipatiaka' caused by vitiation by all three 'doshas', as well as by external factors like poisoning or demonic possession.

'Pancha karma' is the traditional treatment for 'unmaad' (Sarngadhara Samhita; Sect. 3; Chaps. 1 and 3). Ayurveda's preferred method of removing extra 'dosha' and 'ama' (toxins) from the body and psyche is 'pancha karma'. There are three stages to the process. The first is a 'purvakarma', or period of preparation, during which extra 'dosha' and 'ama' are dissolved and sent back to the digestive system by a process of internal and external oleation. Following purgation, which eliminates 'pitta dosha' and reduces anger, resentment and irritability, and emesis, which eliminates excess 'kapha' and lessens depression, grief, and attachment, the next step entails five activities to remove the poisons that have collected in the body. As per Charaka Samhita (Van Loon, 2002), the recovery stage, known as 'praschat karma', is when the digestive fire, 'agni', is carefully watched over and maintained as strong. After that, the body goes through a phase of rejuvenation called 'rasayana', during which the fluid tissues are rebuilt. When the heart, senses, head and bowels are evacuated with the cleaning therapies, the patient achieves mental tranquilly, memory and consciousness, as described in the Charaka's description of 'pancha karma' treatment.

6.6.6.4 Treatment of 'Manodosha' and 'Vyadhis' (Mental Disorders)

The first step to regaining mental clarity is to master the senses and counteract the endless force of desire. In general, sensory impressions that are balancing to 'vata' will be grounding and relaxing; cooling for 'pitta' and supporting the development of compassion; exciting for 'kapha' and supporting for the development of equanimity and mental health (Frawley, 2011). In general, 'manodosha' and 'vyadhis' (mental disorders) are treated as follows (Tripathi, 2001): Strong elimination and alleviation therapies must be used in accordance with the specific requirements of the condition 'manasvyadhi'. Specific mantras (chantings etc.) will be helpful in addition to oral medication when such 'manasrogas' (mental diseases) are connected to exogenous—extrinsic or external causative elements—combined with intrinsic or internal medicaments. These and other 'manas' treatments are nothing more than requirements for the patient to uphold certain moral principles. There are two categories into which all 'manasvyadhis' fall: '**Daivavyapashraya**' and '**Yuktivyapashrayachikitsa**' (Charaka Samhita Sutrasthan, 11/54). Charaka spiritual therapy and psychic therapy are two of the three forms of therapies that are linked to 'manasvyadhis'.

Psycho-Ayurvedic medicines to cure mind and mental disorders abound, and many have their roots in the material potentials. They can be divided into three categories: those that relieve 'vata-dosha' (nervous system), or 'pitta-dosha' (blood circulation system), or 'kaphadosha' (lymphatic system). These contemporary terminologies translate the ambiguous Ayurvedic words. When there are 'vata' signs and symptoms, it doesn't matter what the mental state or 'manasroga' may be. A person will frequently dance, yell out loud, laugh, make varied movements and become emaciated, to name a few characteristics. For these people, internal oleation with sesame oil ('snehana') and external 'abhyanga' (massage) with the same oil or another specially made oil with comparable characteristics (e.g., Narayana Tail etc.) are essential. In addition to this, it is advised to take a mild purgative or laxative ('shodhana'), such as castor oil. Following this body-cleansing procedure for 'vatadosha', some vata-pacifying medications are required (Kumar & Chaudhari, 2016). One can also consult original Ayurvedic texts like the Charaka Samhita for signs, symptoms and remedies for 'pittaj' and 'kaphaj' 'manasroga'. So, Ayurveda, the science of life, encompasses not only medical knowledge but also 'adhyatma' and the strong connections between the mind and health.

Mental toxicity and digestive fire play a vital role in understanding and treating mental disorders. The mental clarity that leads to knowledge, understanding, comprehension, recognition and identity is determined by the digesting capacity of the 'sadhaka pitta' (grey matter of the brain) and 'manas' (sensory mind) (Lad, 2006). Thoughts and emotions have the capacity to feed the intelligence, but 'sadhaka pitta' must first process them (Lad, 2006). The strength and brilliance of the central fire in the stomach and small intestine determine the condition of '**manas agni**', or the capacity of the mind to digest. This is the principal source of heat in the body, and as a result, it ignites the digestive fire of the tissues and cells, supporting the efficient operation of the digestive system of the mind (Lad, 2006). The physical digestion of food and the mental digestion of information have a mystical connection, according to Lad (2006). The build-up of unprocessed sensory information, together with memories, ideas and emotions, can turn into mental poisons when mental digestion is poor or inconsistent (Lad, 2006). The mental 'ama' (channels of the mind) become clogged by these toxic indigestions of thoughts, feelings and emotions, which leads to psychological issues (Lad, 2006). Ayurvedic medicine outlines many remedies for inefficient digestion that can be used to treat that mental toxicity.

6.6.6.5 Ayurveda and Personality

According to Ayurveda, the five 'mahabhutas': 'akasa', 'vayu', 'tejas', 'ap' and 'prithvi' are the building blocks of all living things on earth, including the non-living. These five elements make up both the earth and organism. The three humours of 'vata', 'pitta' and 'kapha' are formed by the combination of these five elements (also called as the 'tridoshas' in unison). Samkhyan philosophy serves as a major inspiration for Ayurvedic concepts. The three 'doshas' are regarded in Ayurveda as being fundamental principles that govern all facets of material creation, including the mineral, plant and animal realms. The 'doshas' have been linked to systems theory in physics, giving this Ayurvedic idea a strong theoretical foundation. 'Prakruti' may be used to link phenotypes and genotypes in the human population, according to preliminary research (Walia & Singh, 2018).

'Guna'-based Personality Types: As discussed earlier in Charaka and Shushruta sections the 'guna'-based personality types include seven types of 'sattvika', six types of 'rajasika', and three types of 'amasika'. Different 'sattvika' kinds have been described as-

1. **Brahma**: The Brahma type people are unadulterated one who is free of passion and enmity, and they are equal to all other beings. These traits are associated with emotional stability in the person.
2. **Arsa**: The main features include sacrifices, studies, vows, and celibacy. The qualities that distinguish people are intelligence and creativity.
3. **Aindra**: These groups include daring, outgoing, and happy-go-lucky people. The mention of women's companionship for the purpose of pleasure, especially in the Sattvika kind of category, is an exception to this rule.
4. **Yamya**: The characteristics are described as being action-ready, unattached, and akin to the God of Death.
5. **Varuna**: Those that possess this trait cluster tend to be reserved and conservative. They are brave and tidy.
6. **Kauvera**: Since the Kauvera is a God of Wealth, those who exhibit these attributes enjoy luxury goods and enjoy leisure time.
7. **Gandharva**: The most common characteristics of people are their love of singing, dancing, and music.

The wrathful disposition predominates in ***Rajasika kinds***. The six types are briefly listed.

1. **Asura**: These people are fierce, cunning, and dishonest.
2. **Raksasa**: The defining traits are intolerance, gluttony, and excessive sleeping.
3. **Paisacha**: These types are known for their love of women, their gluttonous habits, and their cowardice.
4. **Sarpa**: Some of the distinguishing characteristics are quick thinking and courage in unleashing horror.
5. **Praita**: They are very greedy and have an enormous appetite. Untrained characteristics may also present.
6. **Sakuni**: These people tend to be group dependent, tense, and passionately attached.

Tamasika are classified as follows:

1. **Pasava**: They are less educated, sleep more, and engage in excessive sex.
2. **Matsya**: This trait cluster's defining characteristic is its instability. They have a fiery personality and are passionate.
3. **Vanaspati**: Such a person should be regarded as Vanasaptya akin to the plant. Such people lack intelligence and depend on their group.

6.6.6.6 Mental Digestion and Ayurveda

According to Sankhya philosophy, the main evolutions engaged in the process of mental digestion are one's own intelligence ('buddhi'), ego ('ahamkara'), and mind ('manas') (Roger, 2013). The sensory impressions transmitted by the five senses are taken in by, organized by, and stored by the mind. The impressions are then metabolized by intellect, which acts as the digestive fire of the mind, and transformed into experiences and memories (Frawley, 2011). When intellect is working properly, it encourages the environment's 'sattvika' qualities to be absorbed and the 'rajasika' and 'tamasika' ones to be rejected. In this way, the mind exemplifies 'sattvika' qualities like calmness, clarity and generosity while sustaining a healthy balance of 'rajas' and 'tamas' to encourage active participation in life while maintaining deep repose. One's deep consciousness is where one preserves the events and memories that the intelligence creates via its metabolic activities ('chitta'). According to Frawley (2011), this phase of mental digestion is comparable to food that has been digested and has integrated into the physical body. Similar to how the three 'gunas' have been ingested, consciousness has been infused with a ratio of those properties (Frawley, 2011).

To have a better understanding of mental digestion we need to re-examine the concept of 'doshas'. After long discussion of the three 'doshas', the 'subdoshas' that govern mental function should also be discussed. The four 'vata subdoshas' that affect mental health (Moore, 2018) are: 'apana vayu', 'prana', 'udana' and 'vyana'. The evolution of consciousness into perception, sensations, feelings, thoughts and, lastly, emotions is governed by the 'prana vayu' (Lad, 2002). It affects mental health and cognitive function (Lad, 2002). 'Prana' moves the mind (Lad, 2002) and links 'buddhi' (intelligent self) and body; it promotes action and decision-making (Moore, 2018). The regulation of the senses by 'prana vayu' causes the arousal of desire and the quest for sensory experiences. Pure consciousness is the state of motionless 'prana', which is devoid of desire and aversion (Lad, 2002). 'Udana vayu', which controls upward motion, is concentrated in the diaphragm and throat. It stimulates memory and affects how 'manas', or the mind, and 'buddhi', or human intelligence, express emotion. It retains the mind and keeps the mind and body moving at a consistent speed, connecting the mind and body, according to 'vyana vayu', which is located in the heart (Moore, 2018). The lower abdomen is where 'apana vayu' is located, and it controls the evacuation of waste, keeping the body and mental channels clear of poison and obstacles (Moore, 2018). 'Sadhaka pitta' is the 'pitta subdosha' and promotes the transition of sensations into feelings and emotions by introducing the fire element into mental thinking (Lad, 2002). It processes emotions and is found both in the heart and in the grey matter of the brain. It is in charge of transforming sensations into truth and reality, and reality into feelings and memory (Moore, 2018). The component of intelligence known as 'sadhaka' is what gives people a sense of their own uniqueness ('ahamkara'). When the 'sadhaka' is in good shape, our experiences are quickly transformed into knowledge and understanding, which are then stored by the 'tarpaka kapha'. 'Tarpaka' and 'avalambaka' ('kapha') are two 'subdoshas' of the 'kapha' that are specifically involved in mental function (Moore, 2018). The brain's white matter, where 'tarpaka kapha' is largely found, is where memories are stored (Lad, 2002). 'Tarpaka kapha' is where thoughts travel, where they can either be recorded and remembered or released. According to Moore (2018), it nourishes and offers knowledge to 'buddhi' (intellect) and aids people in drawing lessons from their experiences. 'Avalambaka kapha' promotes courage for moral behaviour and is largely found in the heart, lungs and spine. This ‘subdosha’ is linked to compassion, love and support (Lad, 2002). It holds emotions until they are transported by ‘vata’ to the ‘sadhaka pitta’ for processing, uniting the body, mind and intellect (Moore, 2018). So, in summary, the ‘vata subdoshas’ control awareness, perception, expression, integration of the mind and body and waste disposal. The metabolization of experience is governed by the ‘pitta subdosha’. ‘Kapha ‘subdoshas’ also enable the storage of memories and bravery. To coordinate mental digestion, these ‘subdoshas’ communicate with the deep consciousness, intelligence, mind and ego (Labbe-Watson, 2020).

According to the Ayurvedic paradigm, mental indigestion is brought on by an imbalance of the ‘doshas’ (‘vata’, ‘pitta’, and ‘kapha’) or of the mental constitution, which is made up of ‘sattva’, ‘rajas’ and ‘tamas’ (Svoboda, 2004). A vital component of mental digestion is the health of the digestive fire (‘agni’), which is connected with the operation of the ‘doshas’ and the mental ‘gunas’. Six stages make up the pathophysiology of doshic imbalance: accumulation, aggravation, overflow or spreading, depositing, manifestation and diversification (Lad, 2002; Svoboda, 1999). ‘Rajas’ and ‘tamas’ may be out of balance from birth as a result of antenatal, genetic, or karmic influences, or imbalance may happen later in life as a result of vitiating circumstances (Frawley, 2011). ‘Sattva’, which stands for equilibrium, tranquillity and so on, is never the root of mental imbalances. The weak or deficient feeling of ‘ahankara’ (feeling of I) is what first encourages ‘pragyaparadha’ or crimes against knowledge, despite the fact that there are many other factors that contribute to mental imbalance and are listed in both classical and contemporary writings. As per Svoboda (1999), one may swallow more than one can chew if one lets ‘ahamkara’s’ interest in one’s fictitious character control one’s life. There is a chance to vomit unprocessed experience to stop it from entering one’s system. When someone deliberately or unintentionally fails to behave in accordance with the rhythms of nature because desire is present, this is a crime against wisdom. Through desire or attachment, rage, greed, bewilderment, pride, jealousy, repulsion, or fear, a malformed ego can generate imbalances (Lad, 2006). These can appear in a variety of ways, including eating the incorrect foods, being overly active, excluding oneself from nature, permitting the sensory organs and their objects of perception to be in improper connections, and suppressing one’s natural urges (Svoboda, 2004). Other external factors that contribute to imbalance include exposure to pollutants, the negative effects of medical treatment, travelling at fast speeds and picking up other people’s negativity (Svoboda, 2004).

‘Pragyaparadha’ are actions that people take that are not fitting for their nature or circumstance at the time. Such actions typically impair digestion, which promotes the production of ‘ama’, or toxic waste. The physiological and mental channels are no longer conducive to the appropriate flow of ‘vata’ and ‘prana’ after the obstructive ‘ama’ has been introduced into the system (Svoboda, 2004). Even though pathogenic processes can happen in the absence of ‘ama’, nevertheless, it can speed up and aggravate the illness process.

6.6.6.7 Diet, Nutrition and Mental Health

Eating has a bigger impact on bodies and minds than anything else people do. When food is consumed, the body will separate it into its fundamental nutrients (protein, fat, vitamins and minerals) and nuances ('rajas', 'tamas' and 'sattva'). Individual literally becomes what he consumes through the processes of digestion, absorption, and cellular metabolism. It makes sense that the Ayurvedic approach to treating mental illness emphasizes the significance of eating a diet that is both nutritionally sound and suitable for the patient's body's constitution. Frawley (1997) claims that 'rajasika' and 'tamasika' diets upset or dull the mind, induce restlessness and lead to sickness. In contrast, a sattvic diet assists in the treatment of mental problems since it enables the mind to regain harmony and balance. The vegetarian, plant-based 'sattvika' diet emphasizes whole foods. Fresh, top-notch, healthy and organic foods like whole grains and vegetables make up 'sattvika' cuisine. Foods that are processed, canned, bagged, boxed and which lack the life-force energy ('prana') are 'tamasika'. One should avoid eating any foods that might have been obtained by injuring animals, including meat, fish and seafood Frawley (1997). Modern experts also are beginning to recognize how crucial nutrition is in the treatment of mental disease. Research reveals that nutrition not only matters with regard to the problems treated within many medical disciplines, but also has the ability to alter mental outlook and mental disorders, according to review studies in the developing subject of nutritional psychiatry, Nobody can dismiss this, especially in light of the growing evidence that poor mental health and heightened stress appraisals are the root causes of harmful eating behaviours (Logan & Felice, 2014).

6.7 Upanishads

The Samkhya school, one of the schools of Indian philosophy, emphasizes the ideas of 'sattva', 'rajas' and 'tamas'. The themes are also covered in the Vedas and the Bhagvad Gita. Choosing a certain school of thinking is thus one of the conflicts. The explanations given by other literature can be used to refine the Upanishadic concepts of 'sattva', 'rajas' and 'tamas'. Additionally, it can present a chance to create an integrated understanding of 'sattva', 'rajas' and 'tamas'.

6.7.1 'Triguna' and Personality Thoughts in Various Upanishads

Suneeta and Shrikrishna (2009) completed a research review of the 'Triguna' theory and personality thoughts found in various Upanishads, and the study is summarized here. In the **Chhandogya Upanishad** three 'gunas' are indicated by the three colours:

White ('satoguna'), red ('rajoguna') and black ('tamoguna'). The 'guna' 'sattva' is indicated here as in the sense of Nature, not as goodness as described in Sakhyan philosophy. The **Shvetastar Upanishad** also has descriptions of these three colours. Further, this Upanishad shows the primary purpose of the work ('karma'). In the **Katha Upanishad** the senses are described as the lowest or outer part of the body; 'manas' (mind) is higher than the senses; above 'manas' is 'sattva'; above 'sattva' is 'buddhi' (intelligence), and above 'buddhi' is the 'avakya' (unmanifest) (David, 1978). The **Maitri Upanishad** describes the soul ('atman'/Self) in the third chapter. This is the subject of the qualities (gunas)—'sattva', 'rajas' and 'tamas'. Being overcome by the 'gunas', the individual becomes confused, self-conceited, suffers and reincarnates. The **Maitri Upanishad** outlines the characteristics of the 'gunas'. Hume (1962) says with these qualities the elemental soul is overcome and that is why it undergoes various forms:

Dark Qualities ('Tamas'): Delusion, fear, despondency, sleepiness, worriedness, heedlessness, old age, sorrow, hunger, thirst, wretchedness, anger, atheism, ignorance, jealousy, cruelty, stupidity, shamelessness, religious neglect, pride and inequality, among others.
Passionate Qualities ('Rajas'): Inner thirst, affection, emotion, covetouness, maliciousness, lust, hatred, secretiveness, envy, instability, unsteadfastness, fickleness, distractedness, ambitiousness, acquisitiveness, favouritism towards friends, dependence upon surroundings, hatred in regard to unpleasant object of the sense, over-fondness with regard to pleasant objects, sourness of utterance, and gluttony, among others.
Perfect Yogi: In the sixth chapter of the Maitri Upanishad it outlines the characteristics of the perfect yogi: pure, clean, void, tranquil, breathless, selfless, endless, undecaying, steadfast, eternal, unborn, and independent, among others (Suneeta & Shrikrishna, 2009).

The 'Trigunas' (Three Qualities) and their Measurement: Several studies have concentrated on examining the ideas of 'sattva', 'rajas' and 'tamas'. These Vedic notions have also been the subject of research inquiry around the globe, and it appears that they have cross-cultural applicability. This can be shown in the 'trigunas' inventory that was created and published in the journal *Psychological Reports* (Wolf, 1996, 1999). Although it does not compare to the volume of study relating to the yoga school of thinking or that of psychological aspects of the Buddhist school of thought, the 'trigunas' appear to have drawn Indian psychologists from an early era. As a result, nine tests have been created to research the ideas of 'sattva', 'rajas', and 'tamas' (Manickam, 2005). The Samkhya school of thought is the foundation for the ideas that Mohan and Sandhu (1986) investigated. Wolf (1999) developed the instrument specifically on the Vedic philosophy, while Das (1991) made it unique to the Bhagvad Gita. All of the aforementioned instruments were either scales or inventories, but Mathew (as reported by Manickam, 2005). created a Q-sort technique to evaluate 'tamas', 'rajas', and 'sattva'.

The three ideas were viewed by Mathew (2001) in a different way than they were by the Samkhya school of thinking. Mathew (2001) thought that, contrary to popular belief, 'tamas' is not inferior to 'rajas'. Inertia, activation and stability were operationally defined by Mathew, however these definitions don't match the 'tamas', 'rajas', and 'sattva' notions that are mentioned in the Indian conceptions. The relative prominence of these three traits in a person is assessed using the IAS rating scale (Mathew, 1994). Various subscales or variables were proposed by Mathew (1994) and are the result of his years of independent investigation and research. These ideas are mostly related to the 'manomaya' or 'anandamaya koshas', according to a detailed study (Manickam, 2005). Additionally, it has been noted that some of the interpretations of Indian thinking made by later philosophers and psychologists changed the original ideas' original intent. Therefore, it makes sense to accept the original concepts, to regard them as the foundation, and to assimilate knowledge from different schools of thought, which is complementary and clarifies any disparities, without compromising the concepts' original meaning.

6.7.2 The 'Kosha' Theory

Unlike the definition of a person mentioned in the **Taittiriya Upanishad**, some Indian scholars have adopted a different concept of a person. Basu (2001) proposed integral psychology, based on the ideas of Sri Aurobindo. From two perspectives, Basu had two ideas of the person or personality. According to the first, a person is seen as a series of concentration rings in sheaths arrayed as the outer being, inner being and inmost being. However, this viewpoint ignores other crucial aspects of the person mentioned in the Taittirya Upanishad. According to Sri Aurobindo's second idea (as cited by Basu, 2001), the outer being is what is known as personality in psychology and is composed of the physical, vital and mental planes of consciousness, entangled with one other although possessing unique qualities. The ego is the centre of the outer existence. The ego, often known as 'I', is a fictitious construct made from elements of our nature, including the mind, life force, and physical body. The inner being cannot be arranged around the ego; instead, it requires the backing of a *beyond ego* principle.

The **Taittirya Upanishad** defines the five dimensions' functions of psychology of personality:

1. '**Annamaya Kosha**': This sheath could be used to conceptualize the majority of biological processes that are now covered by physiological psychology, with the exception of the psychophysical functions that are a part of pranamaya sheath.
2. '**Pranamaya Kosha**': This sheath may include the psychological and physiological processes as well as sensuous ones.
3. '**Manomaya Kosha**': The functions of the three 'koshas' of 'pranamaya', 'manomaya', and 'vijnanamaya' encompass the majority of the psychological processes that modern psychologists regard to be a component of psychology.
4. '**Vijnanamaya Kosha**': Intelligence is a component of the 'vijnanamaya kosha' which makes it difficult to investigate intelligence as a concept. The results of

modern psychological research on general intelligence, emotional intelligence, and spiritual intelligence may support the idea that intelligence is hierarchical and may also support the connection of the Indian concept of the individual.

5. '**Anandamaya Kosha**': This sheath includes the idea of 'moksha', as well as the functions that are regarded as spiritual in contemporary psychological studies. It is challenging to assign the thoughts to the appropriate type of 'kosha', however, because the Upanishads don't offer a clear-cut prescription for doing so and because of the crucial concept of connectedness (Manickam, 2005).

The Koshas and Personality: According to the **Taittirya Upanishad**'s integrative notion of person, the person is made up of five sheaths (as discussed earlier) or dimensions called the 'annamaya', which are more closely related to the physical. Breathing is tied to the body and is called 'pranamaya'. Mental mechanisms, sentiments and emotions are called 'manomaya' and are related to the mind, 'vijnanamaya', and the last, 'anandmaya' are both connected to knowledge and higher cognitive processes,. Because the 'koshas' or sheaths and 'mahabhutas' are interconnected, everything that affects 'brahman' or the world can also affect the 'atman', and vice versa. The five 'koshas' are not autonomous. These 'koshas' are interconnected despite having their own distinct entities. The balance of all the other dimensions is likely to be impacted by changes in one of these dimensions. The deep, subjective perception of the self is unattainable when one is fully immersed in the outer sheaths (Rao, 1997). The Taittirya Upanishadic idea of person has gained widespread acceptance among Indian psychologists. In the list below, 'koshas' are discussed in a personality psychological perspective:

1. **'Annamaya Kosha'** relates to the physical body's anatomy and physiology. This 'kosha' is responsible for the individuality of the human body's structure, including all physiological systems and their operations.
2. **'Pranamaya Kosha'** relates to the breath, and to the psychological and physical foundations of life. The existence of sensation can only be perceived because the 'prana' stimulates the experience of sensation. Although the sense organs are not included in this 'kosha', they are related to the main purposes of the sense organs.
3. **'Manomaya Kosha'** has to do with the mind, psyche and mental processes. This is a component of the person's psychical system and a sensory tool. This psychical component needs to be functioning for 'prana' to work. 'Manas' is active while awake and while dreaming, but not while deeply asleep. The physiological processes involving the sense organs are not influenced by 'manas'. However, sensations cannot be felt without 'manas' being activated.
4. **'Vijnanamaya Kosha'** relates to knowledge, intellect, and consciousness This 'kosha', which is connected to cognitive processes, is the repository for 'sanskaras', or previous experiences. It is also filled with 'vasanas', or predisposition. The alteration of 'vijnana' occurs as it processes the cognition. The entire person, who includes all the 'koshas', is the perceiver, not just the 'vijnana'.
5. **'Anandamaya Kosha'** means spiritual or beyond. The concept of 'ananda' refers to something that is illogical or incomprehensible. At its functional level, the

other components of the person, which are contained in various sheaths, dissolve. Physical sensations, senses, intellect and 'vijnana' are only a few of the functions that cease to exist. At this level, neither ideation nor intelligence work.

6.8 Jyotisha, Vastu Shastra and Shamudrik Shastra

6.8.1 Jyotisha (Indian Astrology)

The old Hindu astrological system is known as Jyotisha (from the Sanskrit 'jyotia', from 'jyoti' meaning light, heavenly body), or as Hindu astrology, Indian astrology, or more recently Vedic astrology. 'Hindu astrology', as the English translation of 'jyotia' has been in use from the early nineteenth century, although Vedic astrology is a comparatively new phrase, becoming popular with self-help books on related subjects.

Despite not being strong scientific research, astrology aids one in assessing a horoscope's strengths and weaknesses, especially when mental ailment and weakness are combined. This supports the bolstering of a person's weak parts during the formative years, especially if the parents are aware of the specific combinations that require more care and support as the children mature. The three main planetary bodies that control a person's cerebral hemisphere are the Moon ('Chandra'), Mercury ('Budha') and Venus ('Sukra'). The Moon specifically signifies mental nutrition; a poorly placed moon makes the horoscope feeble. Mental fortitude and a healthy imagination can both benefit from a well-fed mind. Mercury influences the neurological system and the respiratory system in the body, as well as the capacity of the brain to retain information and the activity of its nerve centres. Venus is the planet of love, and when it is ill, it can cause love to become irrational and trigger animal tendencies. Unfulfilled desires might cause mental disorders or inappropriate energy outbursts. These three planets, together with the fifth house, play a significant part in astrology and mental illnesses when they are most severely afflicted (Deekshitulu, 2019).

Carl Jung: One of main topics that Jung looked into was astrology, which is a good illustration of an archetype and the collective unconscious. It is an illustration of an archetype in which individuals can distinguish images of stars and planets by their placements. Jung attempted to establish a correlation between events in people's lives and their birth charts using astrology but was unsuccessful. Although Jung and Vastu both examine astrology, they do it in very different ways. The distinction is that Vastu emphasizes the importance of astrology. Hindus produce birth charts that show the planets' positions at the time of birth, just as Jung did with his natal charts (Karani, 2014).

Mental Disorders and Indian Astrology: There are many mental disorders, but common ones, which many people experience, are anxiety, phobias and OCD with varying degrees of severity, while some may experience phobias, schizophrenia, or other disorders that can cause major issues if not addressed in a timely manner.

According to the degree of the moon's weakness in the horoscope, poor upbringing, or a lack of sufficient care during the formative years would undoubtedly have an impact on developing mental disorders (Balaji Deekshitulu, 2019). The Moon is a symbol of the mind. Mercury is in charge of the brain's ability to govern nerves and communication. The Fourth and Fifth Houses are significant ones. Leo and Cancer are important omens. In contrast to transit afflictions, which can pertain to short-term disturbances, natal afflictions to the relevant planets, houses and signs can cause psychiatric disorders and mental problems to remain active for extended periods of time. 'Panchamsa' is the fifth division in the divisional chart for depression (Balaji Deekshitulu, 2019). The Fifth House represents depression. The Fifth House and and the Moon represents peace of emotions. The Fourth House and the Moon represents mental peace. Mercury and the Sixth house represent nervous control. Jupiter is the general 'karaka' (significator) for the Fifth House. The Moon and Venus is the general 'karaka' (significator) for the Fourth House (Balaji Deekshitulu, 2019).

Treatments of Mental Disorders: By doing worship or wearing diamonds, one can strengthen the Lagan Lord. Furthermore, one can offer adoration to the Lagan Lord and any allied deities, don the Moon Yantra, give a silver elephant as donation and worship the evil planet. These are some practices described in Indian astrology to calm the mind and deal with mental health issues. A weak Moon is a major cause of mental disorders and imbalances as per Indian astrology. The Moon brings happiness and calm into one's life. It was discovered that some persons also had weak Moons, and in those circumstances, the person was found to be experiencing issues with their mind, as well as more frequent irritability. Here are several treatments one should try to strengthen the weak Moon in his or her 'kundali'. To reap the most rewards, meditate frequently, particularly in the moonlight. Give white clothing to those in need. Put on a silver 'kada'. Monday fasting helps the Moon grow stronger (Balaji Deekshitulu, 2019). According to Bhawaan's explanation (Tatavarthy, 2007), Clinical Astrology is a branch of Medical Astrology that tries to develop good personalities, improve emotional regulation and address relevant behavioural issues in people. The mental and emotional characteristics shown by the birth chart provide a significant hint for the diagnosis of the majority of ailments. Exercises help one become physically stronger, prayers help one to become mentally stronger inside, and astrology helps one to gain confidence in nature and deity. All diseases stem from a lack of faith and beliefs. Ayurveda focuses on treating physical disorders, but Medical Astrology addresses the underlying reasons, such as psychological and mental imbalances, and fosters a strong faith in the cosmos's natural order. Astrologers contend that by examining a planet's house position and the impact of other planets on the governing planet of a chart, it is possible to make astrological predictions (Balaji Deekshitulu, 2019).

6.8.2 Vastu Shastra (Traditional Hindu Architecture)

Vastu refers to the study of how a house is built, the collective or totality of energies and powers that become a reality as a result of the private structure's geometry, shape, and scale, the materials used in its construction, and its dynamic interactions with the environment (Sundaravadivelu, 2013). Structures can and should work with nature's forces rather than against them, making the person an important component of the area or situation. Layers of atmospheres or vitality levels exist within the human body. The improvement of the individual determines how well these vitality levels are. When the essential fields of the individual and the vital fields of the structure connect, both good and bad outcomes follow. Making a home with the intention that the two vitality levels: one of the animate and the other of the lifeless, work together and in resonance is, therefore, much more crucial. The purpose of the general grandiose vitality emanating from the divine bodies or planets is to minimize the evil energies and maximize the magnificent energies at different stages of development. It is remarkable that living things experience direct and indirect effects of immeasurable vitality (Sundaravadivelu, 2014). In this case, the various surrounding energies might be arranged in such a way as to positively resonate with the person or people residing in the building, giving their lives significance and harmony. Therefore, the various creative, hazardous and ongoing energies that are present in the cosmos as described in the Vastu Shastra must be researched.

Vastu Shastra and Carl Jung's views: It can be seen that Jung studied both Buddhism and Hinduism in order to comprehend Eastern religions. Vastu Shastra does not mention archetype, although it contains ideas that are comparable to it. This is in contrast to how Jung defines archetype. The connection is in Carl Jung's description of the archetype as an invariable nucleus of meaning, which only exists in concept and not in actuality (Jung, 1999). When describing an archetype's traits, that particular entity is kept apart. The archetype of a mother, for instance, is real in theory, but when it comes to comprehending a mother, she is far more complex than just being a mother. Humans have both a good and a bad side, much like the universe and Vastu mentions particular deities. This connects to Jung's idea that it's important to accept the dark side. Psychological repression, which can result from not accepting this negative side, may be at the root of some psychological problems. In order to create positive environments, Vastu Shastra uses both the positive and negative sides of the concerned worshipping or authoritative deities.

According to Vastu, a mandala is an 81-square cosmological grid that symbolizes the might of either a god or goddess. This grid is condensed to a simple grid of nine squares. The Vastu Purusha is restrained and held in place by all of these gods and goddesses. If the devil were to manifest, he would wreak havoc on everyone who lived there. The mandala serves two purposes: first, to inspire the design of a physical space, and second, to reveal the artist's psyche. Although both Vastu and Jung mention the word 'mandala', they both refer to it as a metaphor for the cosmos (Karani, 2014). Both terms refer to the features of the universe that cannot be seen and how these aspects affect our daily life. The difference is that Vastu employs it to link the occupant of the space with the forces of the universe, whereas Jung uses it largely to study and grasp the totality of Self (Karani, 2014). Jung utilized it to analyze the drawn mandala and gain insight into his own and his patients' inner struggles. The individual who was attempting to be understood would create the mandala. Jung would first meditate to get to the place where he could draw a mandala. The act of meditating would liberate the subconscious from the ego, enabling the mandala to serve as a symbol of the inner struggle. Mandalas are used by Vastu Shastra to map the energy of the universe onto a surface. The architect can then place the various functionalities in the relevant zones once the basic grid has been set up. According to Vastu Shastra, there are three layers of energies: the subconscious, the physical environment and the cosmos. The inner self is at ease and generates positivity by drawing a mandala and using it as the framework for a strategy.

According to Jung, the concept of god in religion is an example of a spiritual archetype since it is an image that its adherents are familiar with. However, according to Vastu, if the gods and goddesses are content, their devotees will live happy and prosperous lives. According to Vastu, gods and goddesses are natural energies that must be balanced in order to produce positive places. The powers were referred to as gods and goddesses, and their wrath was emphasized so that the tradition was not questioned in order for the average devotees to adhere to the Vastu regulations (Karani, 2014). In his search for the ultimate reality, Jung spoke of spiritual things in terms of the higher Self, or the inner world of the soul. Hinduism considerss that the soul's union with god is its ultimate goal. Jung disagreed with this idea since it implied that the soul would cease to exist if it united with god (Karani, 2014). Vastu and Jung both research the spiritual or intangible components of the material and physical worlds. Both make an effort to respond to inquiries about subconscious experiences. Jung would likely discuss the psychological implications of the archetypes of the house, family, mother and father, among other things, or urge the users to make mandalas to better understand their emotions, among other things. The mandala generates energies that affect how the user feels the space, and the mandala created by the individual is a way to understand how the subconscious is affected by the home. Both are genuine attempts to comprehend the user's experience. Similar to Jung's ideas about balancing opposites in life, Vastu Shastra relies on balancing the energy of the home. Jung took up yoga in an effort to detach from his ego and find peace. The Vastu Shastra advises individuals who adhere to it to practise yoga regularly at home. The person's chakras open up as they practice yoga. This results in alignment of the inner self, the house and the spiritual. People who reside in a home with proper Vastu will feel positive energy, making it possible for them to meditate or engage in yoga. While Jung was unaware of the influence astrology may have on people's lives, Vastu heavily utilizes it. The birth chart of the home's owner is created, and a number of fortunate times are determined based on it. Jung employed the mandala, a pattern that architects use to design a positive place, to better understand his own and his patients' psyches. Karani (2014) proposed that, it might be a way for architects and psychiatrists to collaborate and comprehend how individuals are affected by built environments.

6.8.3 Shamudrik Shastra (Body Features Analysis)

The study of face reading, aura reading and full body analysis is known as Samudrik Shastra and is a component of the Vedic tradition. It is also one of the topics that the *Garuda Purana* incorporates. The Sanskrit phrase 'samudrik shastra' approximately translates to knowledge of physical aspects. Since it is connected to astrology, palmistry ('hast-samudrik'), phrenology ('kapal-samudrik') and face reading, it is frequently utilized in Vedic astrology (physiognomy, 'mukh-samudrik') (Fouw & Svoboda, 2003).

Prasad (2012) found three psyches: actual, manifested and construct. These psyches are based on various naturally occurring facial shapes, geometrical features, and architectural aspects of the eyes, with emphasis on the nose, ears, lips, forehead and chin. Because this will assist the prediction validity of the psychological state and dependability of the recognized psyche of a person, statistical criteria Are utilized to distinguish between different psyches. Any manipulation is a sign that the intended individual is the subject of false information. According to Shankhya *philosophy*, Humans are naturally born with certain traits, meaning that the human psyche is unpolluted. The face is a predictor of an individual's true psyche in addition to serving as a symbol of their attractiveness or establishing their identity. Face management is founded in theories of emotion and management skills since people can give and receive both positive and negative feedback. This is merely an erroneous perception of the target person. Numerous predictions have been produced based on emotion research, but these conclusions are only time and situation dependent. A person's predicted characteristics should match their real facial features, which may be impossible in their given emotional state and behaviour. This does not imply that studies of human behaviour that focus on emotions are meaningless. The ability to uncover a person's hidden psyche is a goal of both electronic- (brain-mapping) and pharmacological-based studies on human psyche prediction (Prasad, 2012). This is the narrative of pretty much all psychological discoveries, yet efforts to maximize accuracy and predictability have always drawn psychologists. The work of psychometricians is commendable, and theories of measurement emphasize behaviour prediction. Their degree of restriction might occasionally make decisions risky. This work aims to accurately estimate how a person should be in order to make predictions. There are specific facial feature combinations that can be used to predict the shape of faces. The conceptual truth of face contour also serves as the foundation for the Vedic concept of identifying human nature.

Biometrics: The biometric system has so far been successful in resolving the major identifying and verification issues. However, research being done in these areas is unable to use the current biometric system to fully understand a person's mentality. Given the broad range of applications for biometrics, it is advisable to classify biometrics according to their intended usage. Kumar et al. (2011) divided biometric into three categories. Using various biometric technologies for identification and verification in the current scenario is categorized as Biometric-I. Further, it has been noted since the Vedic period, which dates back to 2,000 BC, that an individual's characteristics can be determined or read by examining the imprints of different human parts, such as the face, hand, ear and so on. This analysis falls within the Biometric-II category. In addition, recently, there has been a lot of studies carried out to determine which diseases a person has by looking at different body parts, which is referred to as Biometric-III. The Vedas claim that the three natural modes, or 'gunas', of 'satva', 'rajas' and 'tamas', are present in all material substances. In Vedantic literature, human beings are frequently described in terms of nine lotus petals and the three characteristics, or 'gunas' (Kumar et al., 2011). The Atharva Veda contains the initial mention. The Big Five model, the most well-known model of psychological characteristics, refers to the aforementioned 'gunas' as openness, conscientiousness, extraversion, agreeableness and neuroticism. The Big Five aspects of personality are five basic personality domains or dimensions in modern psychology, to which we can relate Vedantic 'gunas' and perspectives.

Geometry of the face and the eyes can accurately anticipate a person's concealed psychological condition. For the purpose of this forecast of the individual's psyche, the geometrical output and mathematical presumptions used in statistical computation serve as sufficient indicators of the indicated factors. The mind engineering theory used in this case can forecast enough details about a person's psychological reality in both an ideal and fostered condition of human psychology. Standard deviation of face geometry status focused on the female status and discovered that it was distinct from the male. High female Standard deviation projected that the female psychology is probably different from the male's. The psychological state of a woman can vary, but that is her true psyche, which depends on the engineering of her face, not their construct or displayed psychology (Prasad, 2012). The necessity to comprehend the psyche inside the geometrical outcome is emphasized by a two-dimensional examination of the facial architecture and related regions of the face, particularly the eyes. By comparing the output of these algorithms to eye tracking data, Privitera and Stark (2000) assessed ten alternative algorithms for detecting regions of interest. They came to the conclusion that it was unrealistic to expect an algorithm to accurately forecast where every zone of interest would be. Eye to ear geometrical output suggests that a particular inherent architecture of the face, which varies between males and females, influences the human mind.

Face Analysis: In terms of Vedic psychology, the function of the face includes speech and the connection between the body and the mind. For character recognition, modern psychology looks at different universal expressions of rage, fear, disgust, melancholy, delight, disdain, surprise and fascination. The index of the mind is the face. It provides information on the person's aptitude and propensities, as well as information about their prior lives and childhood. Vedic face reading's fundamental tenet is that the subtle body, which has been evolving during countless incarnations, lies on top of the gross physical body. The entire body can serve as a source of knowledge in this way. The Vedic work devoted to this topic includes descriptions of some of this (Samudrika Shastra). The face is the most informational area of the body even though the entire body has information since it has the most complicated muscles. There are three basic methods for identifying psychological traits from a face. The first two, *physiognomy* and *phase facial portrait*, evaluate various face aspects; the second, *ophthalmogeometry*, obtains and interprets parameters from the eye region. The third, *physiognomy*, deals with angles of facial features and facial asymmetry. According to the principle of physiognomy, a person's face, facial features, skin condition and other outward physical characteristics can reveal information about their character or personality (Kumar et al., 2011).

According to the Atharva Vedic *Muhasastra*, as described by Kumar et al. (2011), by looking at a person's entire face, one can gain a clear understanding of their traits, from their early years to their older years. The general study of regions, such as the Parents' region, the Career and Success region, the Life region, the Middle Age region, the Love and Emotional region, the Fertility and Children region, and the Old Age region, provides information on the health of the parents and the individual's career prospects. Further these regions explore attitudes toward life, longevity, negative traits, congenital issues, intense emotional investment in romantic relationships, procreation, energy, childlessness, and risks of drowning, poisoning and so forth.. Face shapes like round, square, rectangle, and triangular, as well as straight, concave, and convex faces, indicate laziness, dullness, creativity, humour, fastidiousness, toughness, aggression and offensiveness. They also indicate sociability, a strong physical build, honesty, aptitude for diplomacy and leadership, suitability for jobs as executive and official, anger and temperamental traits like cheerfulness and brilliance, hyperactivity and sensitivity and disturbed behaviour. In order to identify intelligence, opulence enjoyed in life, obstacles encountered in one's career, longevity, broadmindedness, perfection in work, lack of seriousness, prudence, calculative nature and insecure mind, instability and agitation, untrustworthiness, untimely death, cruelty and perversion, inability to hide affections and emotions, secretiveness, extroversion, cynicism and flirtatiousness, one should look at the person's forehead, eyes, colour of eyes, nose, lips, mouth, chin and jaw. In most cases of face analysis (Shamudrik Shastra), determining a person's inner self involves observing their outward appearance.

Eyes' Analysis: The natural structure of the eyes not only reveals a feature of the face but also the person's beauty, vision, and psychology. Diverse eye sizes and shapes serve different purposes in the human brain. Now, this raises the question, how can one specifically identify the eyes in a person's face to determine the status of their mental conditions? Two methods, a mosaic image and a geometrical face model are used to detect eye types (Prasad, 2012). The detection of eye corners as they appear inside the eyes' window is also a requirement for sharp detection; this is done by video coding, pattern recognition, natural texture analysis and classification. Factual dimensions are expanded on this information. One way a person can think, 'I am a winner' and feel, 'I am superior to others' is by controlling their facial and eye expressions. However, the eye has the ability to reflect one's psychology, which is beyond of one's management purview. Sight and motion, the two primary functions of the human eye, reveal a side of the mind that is not seen in the face or eyes. More than any other face feature, it is thought that the eye can convey the mental process (Santon, 2008). The eye test is one of two characteristics that are important predictors of mental character. The eye is more striking than any other aspect of the face, and it also conveys brilliancy and the appearance of an active life. For this journey, eye alignment is helpful. There are two ways to determine how the eyes are aligned. The iris image and retinal image are compared with a recorded image of the iris portion and retinal portion, the stored image matching to eye alignment at a previous period, as the first step in determining the eye alignment. Finding an eye position at which the retinal picture, iris image and stored image are nearly similar is what this initial method entails in more detail. The second method of assessing eye alignment entails establishing a relationship between the imaging system's instrument axis and the subject's eye's axis. More specifically, the papillary axis may be the subject's eye's axis. Understanding the many characteristics of eyes is necessary for the evaluation of the psyche (mind) through the eyes (Prasad, 2012). The eye's form, size, colour, brightness, commissure shape, fold effect, angle of inclination, relative position of central line, and general expression, among others are the study areas relevant to the Shamudrik Shastra and for other predictive purposes.

Hand Analysis: Brain and mind are reflected in palms. The palm lines are a reflection of the relationship between a person's mind and behaviour. Those with the mental and physical capacity to achieve renown can be identified by the flag of fame on their palms. The secondary line supplies energy and potential for a specific mount as the triangle gathers and protects the energy of the lines. This makes a person well-known in a certain field or vocation. Finally, it can assert that the popularity that comes with fame is something that many well-known figures from many walks of life have experienced (Panda, 2019). The ancient Indian sages shared their understanding of the hand, which they acquired via observation, manipulation and analysis. The information gained in this way shed light on every element of existence. The science of hand analysis continued to grow, prosper and find favour in the world of knowledge as it extended to various nations (Katakkar, 1992). Two factors are essential for good hand analysis. The capacity for observation comes first, followed by the capacity for comparing and contrasting various features. A framework for organizing all the hints discovered in a hand is another useful tool in the area of hand analysis. It's crucial to note the order in which each hand's components are dealt with (Collins, 2008). The hand is separated into three zones from the standpoint of hand psychology. The first zone, which is made up of the thumb, the index finger and the space below them, imparts environmental awareness, thoughtful behaviour and willpower. The ring finger, little finger and the area beneath them are all considered to be in the second zone. This area is a reliable predictor of the subconscious mind and a person's hidden traits. The social zone, located in the centre of the zone, represents a person's capacity for social adjustment (Katakkar, 1992). The shape of the hand serves as the foundation for hand science. It should be noted that the shape of the hand plays a significant role in revealing the sort of mind that is controlling the subject's actions in life.

In hand analysis, the elevated fleshy areas are referred to as 'mounts'. They show how different parts of our brain are functioning. They are the magnetic centres that transmit the sub-conscious mind's message in the form of lines. Nine mounts, or divisions of each palm, make up each palm. Each mount reflects the person's unique mental and physical characteristics, such as their level of egoism, extroversion, introversion sympathy, creative ability, patience, and endurance. The analysis of the line can be used to explain how to identify both positive features and the characteristics of different sorts of offenders. The ability to diagnose both mental illness and illness brought on by psychological distress is also very accurate. The heart's line can reveal a person's more ethereal, unfathomable and subtle faculties—the ones that eventually determine their character and personality. The most significant line on the hand is the head line, which represents the brain, mental energies, and intellectual ability. The hand is split in half by this line. The higher portions depict the growth of the mind, while the lower portions display the growth of the body (Kumar et al., 2011). The life line typically depicts a person's vigour and energy. The quantity of the vitality is revealed by the length, depth, and continuity. This line has a strong psychological component as well.

Medical Diagnosis: The AtharvaVeda is one of the four Vedas, along with RigVeda, SamaVeda and YajurVeda. It addresses mental health and sickness through the notion of 'trigunas', which includes 'sattva', 'rajas' and 'tamas'. The face is a mirror of the mind. Physical and mental wellness both may be the signs of how beautiful and well-structured one's face is. The tongue, eyes, nails, varied skin patterns (dermatoglyphics) and hair distribution were once used by doctors to detect disorders. In general, it only involves diagnosing illnesses based on physical signs. The face and hands might give away a person's health status. According to the 'Mishio Kushi' (face reading) theory, acne can develop on specific body parts if an organ or gland is weak or poisonous (Kumar et al., 2011). The brightness of the face is a reliable indicator of the body's wellness. From this point forward, the face and hand can be transformed into a continuum of distinct facial areas, each of which indicates the state of the body's health whether physical or mental.

6.9 Kamasutra and Psychology

According to many Indian scholars the Vatsyayana Rishi was never married and was 'balbrahmchari' (following strict celibacy). Then, how could he write such a tremendous book on sex education? Another example is Adi Jagad Guru Shankarchryta, who was also 'balbrahmachari' and conducted a 'shastrasrtha' (discussion of philosophical theories) with a Mandan Mishra's (Vaishnav Acharya's) wife on the topic of 'kaamshastra' (sex education). And some other achryas (scholars) are further examples of this strange. An ancient Indian Sanskrit treatise on sexuality, eroticism and emotional pleasure in life is known as the Kamasutra (Wendy, 2003). Credited to Vatsyayana (Haksar & Favre, 2011), the Kamasutra was written as a guide to the art of living well, the nature of love, finding a life-mate, preserving one's love life and other aspects relevant to the pleasure-oriented capacities of human life. It is not exclusively or primarily a sex manual on sex positions (Wendy & Sudhir, 2002). It is a text in the 'sutra' genre that has pithy, aphoristic verses that have persisted into the current period with various 'bhasyas' (commentaries). The earliest evidence of attitudes regarding sex is found in the texts of Buddhism, Jainism and Hinduism, the first of which is possibly the oldest piece of literature still in existence. The Vedas, the world's oldest scriptures, present moral viewpoints on sexuality, marriage and reproductive knowledge. The three pillars of Hinduism: 'Dharma', 'Artha', and 'Kama', represent religious obligation, material welfare and sensuous aspects of life, respectively, in Vatsyayana's famous work, Kamasutra, which was composed some time between the first and sixth centuries (Chakraborty & Thakurata, 2013). The expression of the Indian perspective toward sex as a fundamental and natural part of the Indian psyche and way of life seems to be the main focus here (Burton & Arbuthnot, 1984).

6.9.1 *Family Psychology*

According to Upadhyaya (1965), the first verse of the book Kamasutra argues that marriage is a means of fostering a pure and genuine love between the couples. It results in emotional fulfilment in a variety of ways, including the joint pursuit of 'dharma' (spiritual and ethical life) and 'artha' (economy) as well as additional friends and family for both parties, offspring, a romantic and sexual relationship and procreation (Upadhyaya, 1965). The first three chapters cover how a man should go about finding the ideal bride, while the fourth chapter covers a woman's options for finding the proper mate (Upadhyaya, 1965). According to the text, a person needs to be realistic and have the same attributes that one expects from the relationship. It advises involving friends and family in the search and getting to know future spouse's present friends and family before getting married (Upadhyaya, 1965). Alain Danielou (1993) quotes Vatsyayana as saying that one should play, marry and socialize with one's equals, individuals of one's own circle, who share the same principles and worldview. According to Kamasutra (verse 3.1.20), it is more difficult to maintain a good, happy relationship when there are fundamental differences between the two (Danielou, 1993).

6.9.2 *Sex Education*

Vatsyayana's Kamasutra discusses numerous types of intimacy, including that which occurs between lovers prior to and during intercourse. Kama Sutra (Verses 2.2.7–23), for instance, describes eight different types of 'alingana' (embrace): 'sphrishtaka', 'viddhaka', 'udghrishtaka', 'piditaka', 'lataveshtitaka', 'vrikshadhirudha', 'tilatan-dula', and 'kshiranira' (Upadhyaya, 1965). The first four are nonsexual yet indicate a mutual love. The last four embrace styles are ones that Vatsyayana advises using to enhance pleasure during foreplay and intimate moments. The several types of closeness express the desire and offer ways to entice multiple senses for pleasure. For instance, Vatsyayana asserts that the 'lalatika' form allows both parties to feel one another and gives the man the opportunity to see the complete beauty of the female form (Upadhyaya, 1965). 'Chumbanas' (kissing) is another illustration of the kind of closeness the Kamasutra discusses. The literature covers 26 different types of kisses, ranging from those that are suitable for foreplay and sex, to those used to express respect and affection (Upadhyaya, 1965). Vatsyayana also notes regional differences in the customs surrounding kissing in ancient India. According to the Kama Sutra, the finest kiss for a close partner is one that is based on awareness of the 'avastha' (the emotional state of one's partner) while the two are not engaged in sexual activity. The text advises flowing with the flow and mirroring with 'abhiyoga' and 'samprayoga' during intercourse (Upadhyaya, 1965).

6.9.3 Social Psychology

One of the few sources of knowledge available on ancient India's sociology and cultural environment is the Kamasutra. It explains not only sexual education but the way of life for all Varnas people (Brahmin, Kshtriya, Veshya and Sudras) also. It also describes sexual behaviour across various 'Varna' (class) and 'Jati' (caste). In the Kamasutra (as per Wendy, 2016), lovers are described as not upper-class, yet they must be rich enough to dress nicely, engage in social activities, purchase gifts and surprise their partner. The only time caste is mentioned in the book is when a man is advised to tell amusing tales about other virgins of the same 'Jati' (caste) in order to entice a woman. In general, the literature discusses gender-neutral sexual behaviour between men and women in both urban and rural contexts (Wendy, 2016).

There are other examples of indigenous texts indicating and relating sexuality with daily life. The *Panchatantra* claims that only when a creature's stomach is full do they exhibit shyness, friendship, a melodious voice, intelligence, brilliance of youth, enjoyment of a woman's sensuality, equanimity within the species, absence of sorrow or misery, carnal pleasure, religion, scriptures, intelligence of Brihaspathi (the teacher of Gods/Devathas), hygiene and concern for good behaviour. This graceful Subhashitha from Vishnu Sharma's *Panchathanthra* makes it abundantly obvious how important it is to eat well and get enough nutrients in order to be mentally and physically fit for optimal sexual performance (Chakraborty & Thakurata, 2013). The most well-known example of a traditional Islamic sex handbook is *The Perfumed Garden* by Sheikh Nafzawi. What were considered to be the most desirable traits of lovers and romantic behaviour are eloquently and colourfully depicted in this (Burton, 1964).

6.10 Indian Scholars/Saints

6.10.1 Maharishi Mahesh Yogi

Maharishi Mahesh Yogi's contribution (in Vedic psychology) to elucidating the framework of human development is exceptional because, theoretically speaking, he has elaborated the Vedic paradigm of consciousness in a coherent, scientifically systematic and precisely defined sequence of development that leads to the full unfoldment of human potential. The advanced practice programme and the meditation technique, which are consistent with an active lifestyle, easy to use, open to scientific study and promote the entire spectrum of human development, are the second set of systematic and uniform practices he has made available (Maharishi Mahesh Yogi, 1969). The third addition is Maharishi's Vedic psychology, which not only suggests a basic link between humans and nature, but also a theory of human development and methods to cultivate this (Dillbeck & Alexander, 1989). According to ancient Vedic knowledge, the origin of all apparent existence is a single field that has been described as a field of pure intelligence in nature (Maharishi Mahesh Yogi, 1969). This description is quite current. Physics is currently concentrating its efforts on developing a consistent unified field theory, and the key components of such a theory are now in place (Green, 1986). The undivided field of intelligence in nature can be directly experienced by the person and fully unfolded in human existence, which, in the view of Mahesh Yogi's Vedic psychology, makes such a field realistically relevant to human life. The underlying unity of nature becomes completely accessible to experience once human consciousness has reached its full potential, unifying and enhancing all facets of life (Maharishi Mahesh Yogi, 1986).

Mahesh Yogi's Vedic psychology, which is founded on his rebirth of the knowledge discovered in ancient Vedic science, offers a thorough explanation of adult progression to higher levels of consciousness. It lists the seven main mental and emotional states (Dillbeck & Alexander, 1989). The transcendental or pure consciousness state that is experienced during the Transcendental Meditation programmes, as well as three other states of consciousness, each of which constitutes a stable stage of development past the generally accepted endpoint of adult development, are the three changing states of waking, dreaming and deep sleep. These higher stages of consciousness, cosmic consciousness, refined cosmic consciousness and unity consciousness, develop through regular experiences of transcendental consciousness in contrast to routine daily activities. This development of the mind and body is the foundation for these higher stages. According to modern theories of adult development, the emergence of higher states of consciousness can be seen as an extension of growth that goes beyond the levels of (sensorimotor skills) and thought (mental operations and rational processes) (Dillbeck & Alexander, 1989).

Transcendental Meditation: Transcendental Meditation, a silent awake state, is defined as an experience of pure consciousness devoid of any emotions, ideas or senses (Maharishi Mahesh Yogi, 1969). In order to experience pure consciousness, individuals must be in a state of 'Being' rather than thinking, where they are left awake by themselves in complete knowledge of themselves without any perception of an object (Maharishi Mahesh Yogi, 1963). The principles of this model are phenomenologically supported by experiences of pure consciousness while practising Transcendental Meditation. The Transcendental Meditation technique is made for transcending, which is a process of allowing the focus to shift from levels of active thought to quieter levels of mind where self-awareness is paramount, and thoughts are secondary until ultimately disappearing (Maharishi Mahesh Yogi, 1969). Maharishi Mahesh Yogi's *Maharishi Vedic Science* presents and elaborates on both the Transcendental Meditation method and the dynamics of pure consciousness (Maharishi Mahesh Yogi, 1994).

Vedic Psychology of Development: Maharishi's Vedic psychology holds that after the development of the structure typical of normal adult mind, a progressive sequence of transformations in the fundamental structure of knowledge should take place. It describes a progression of higher developmental phases, sometimes known as higher states of consciousness or enlightenment. These conditions signify the comprehensive development of the mind, emotions, and body (Dillbeck & Alexander, 1989). Although it is claimed that the higher phases are potentially accessible to everyone, their realization is uncommon until consciousness is trained through the experiences offered by particular practices that have been passed down from the Vedic tradition (Maharishi Mahesh Yogi, 1969). Maharishi talks about seven states of consciousness of which three are stable higher stages and four are transient states. All people experience the first three transitory states of consciousness: awake, dreaming and dreamless sleep (Maharishi Mahesh Yogi, 1972). The alternating of these primary states of consciousness is said to be the extent of life before the advent of enlightenment. According to Maharishi's Vedic psychology, a person's ability to experience all three levels of consciousness at once is constrained. The united person cannot exhibit their full potential or act spontaneously in a way that serves both their own interests and the interests of others when their consciousness is not in tune with the field of pure intelligence in nature (Maharishi Mahesh Yogi, 1986). The individual repeatedly causes the individual and collective existence to suffer as a result, according to their opinion on nature. From this adult life, only a modest amount of development is expressed.

Higher States of Consciousness: According to Alexander, a higher state of consciousness would satisfy the following conditions: (1) Extend symbolic representation as far beyond the sensory domain as possible from conceptual representational thought; (2) Need significant neurophysiological development; and (3) Remove the primary ontological and epistemological restriction of the level of abstract reasoning, namely; the restriction that the reflective knower cannot directly know itself (Alexander, 1990). Because the sensation of pure consciousness is a real experience during Transcendental Meditation practice, it is possible that there are states of consciousness other than awake, dreaming, and sleeping (Travis, 2018). The concept of higher levels of consciousness presented by Maharishi Mahesh Yogi in his book *Maharishi Vedic Science* serves as the foundation for the discussion (Maharishi Mahesh Yogi, 1994, 1997).

The Fourth State of Consciousness: According to Maharishi, experiencing the Fourth Major State of Consciousness, also known as Transcendental Consciousness or Pure Consciousness (Maharishi Mahesh Yogi, 1972) is the real beginning of development to a higher level of and physiological functioning. The knower experiences the field of consciousness itself in its unadulterated, unbroken wholeness, free from any thought, emotion, or self-referral state of consciousness. This experience is said to be independent of any thought, emotion, or self-referral state of consciousness. That is, all representational systems or categories, including the subject-object relationship, descended (Maharishi Mahesh Yogi, 1972). According to certain theories, unbounded or universal consciousness is the state of pure consciousness. Maharishi's practical method for achieving its effortlessness is distinguished by the person's awareness shifting from a state of activity to a state of quiet while remaining; the mind is not pressed to be still (Maharishi 1969). Maharishi claims that the reason for this is because these subtler or more refined levels of mental activity and consciousness are more enticing or pleasing than other levels of thinking or perception, and, thus, attention can be guided in this direction (Maharishi Mahesh Yogi, 1969).

The Fifth State of Consciousness: Transcendental Consciousness or Pure Consciousness differs significantly from awake, sleeping and dreaming in terms of its experience. A fifth state of consciousness is known as Cosmic Consciousness. Throughout the course of Transcendental Meditation practice, Transcendental Consciousness typically appears for many seconds at a time. Transcendental Consciousness experience starts to be blended with waking, dreaming and sleeping by alternating it with daily life during Transcendental Meditation practice (Frederick, 2021). Now, on a continuum of inner self-awareness, the remaining sleep, fictitious dream imagery and shifting waking sensations come and go (Maharishi Mahesh Yogi, 1969). This condition is referred to as a fifth stage of consciousness in the Vedic tradition, known as 'Turiyatit Chetana' or Cosmic Consciousness (Maharishi Mahesh Yogi, 1997). In Cosmic Consciousness, all activity occurs on the surface of life; utter silence that is unaffected by current experience exists deep inside.

According to Maharishi's Vedic psychology, the fifth level of consciousness is the first of the higher phases of growth since it symbolizes a consistent form of experience. It is the initial stage of permanent enlightenment. The experience of Pure Consciousness serves as the finest metaphor for both the structure of this stage and its developmental process. The quality of waking, dreaming and sleeping states of consciousness are projected to improve with regular experience of Pure Consciousness due to the practice's physiological consequences. That is, it is anticipated that the quality of restful alertness will persist into deep sleep and wakefulness, resulting in an improved level of rest during sleep and higher physiological stability and activity efficacy in the waking state (Maharishi Mahesh Yogi, 1972).

The Sixth and Seventh States of Consciousness: The term 'Refined Cosmic Consciousness', which refers to the sixth level of consciousness in Maharishi's Vedic psychology framework, is an extension of the stage of Cosmic Consciousness. In the development stage of enlightenment, pure consciousness continues to serve as the foundation for the daily cycle of waking, dreaming and deep sleep, as well as the major setting for the enhancement of environmental perception. According to phenomenology, a closing between the Self (pure consciousness) and the object of Mahesh Yogi's 1972 work relates to the development inside perception that takes place with consciousness. With the development of cosmic consciousness, the gap between self and object begins to decrease. In cosmic consciousness, the Self is perceived as distinct from the activity of cognition. The affective experience of then dominated by the most refined emotional qualities, such as love (Maharishi Mahesh Yogi, 1969). On individual gains, neurophysiological functioning is also expected to be followed by a more deeply positive influence on experience quality.

Application of Model of Consciousness: It is possible to use this more comprehensive theoretical model of consciousness in daily life (Frederick, 2021). For instance, it offers a more thorough foundation for rehabilitation than current approaches (Travis, 2015). Behaviour manipulation is the level at which behavioural modification operates. Cognitive behavioural therapy focuses on altering thought patterns in order to alter behaviour (Leahy, 1996). To aid in the promotion of mental and emotional recovery, compassion-focused therapy encourages individuals to grow in compassion for both themselves and others (Gilbert, 2014).

6.10.2 Sri Aurbindo

Sri Aurobindo's perspective (integral psychology) has addressed the nature of reality in general as well as the nature of the self. He described integral yoga, a brand-new school of yoga. He holds that the material world is one manifestation of consciousness, or the Brahman, in its many manifestations. The line between the partial (matter) and the energy (wave form) blurs as one delve deeper. 'Purusa' is the pure consciousness that appears as 'prakruti', or the world as it is. In accordance with Sri Aurobindo's model of personality, every human being possesses two distinct types of consciousness. One type of consciousness is the outward consciousness with which people often interact, and the other type of consciousness is the hidden internal consciousness. Human beings know relatively little about the second type of consciousness. When one does 'Sadhana', the inner consciousness starts to awaken, allowing one to go within and have a different experience as they connect with their true selves. One starts to live more and more from the within out as the Sadhana develops, and the outside world is perceived as something flimsy and extraneous. In this stage, the mind constantly pulls in the direction of unification with the divine, which is the true goal of human existence. It considers consciousness to be a gradient between the lower and higher spiritual planes. It claims that inanimate objects or the conscience contain the lowest type of consciousness. The physical or body consciousness, vital consciousness, and mental consciousness make up the next degree of consciousness, which is that of the inner being. Both animals and humans have a bodily or body consciousness.

The higher cognitive processes, intelligence, and cognition all relate to the inner consciousness. The higher levels of consciousness, above mind, become accessible through Sadhana with the emergence of the psychic being. The psychic entity enlightens us as to why we are here. The ability to handle more concepts at once is a feature of the **higher mind**. The ability to replicate intuition and the realization that knowledge is not the discovery of the unknown are both characteristics of the **intuitive mind**. There is nothing else to learn: the only thing we can learn is about ourselves. The following level is the **over mind**, when a person discovers a larger unity, oneness, and a higher and more comprehensive truth. At this point, everything is connected and orderly. The **super mind** follows the over mind. A universal perspective is the super mind. Once a person is able to communicate with the super mind, it has the power to completely alter that person's nature (Manonmaniam Sundaranar University, n.d.). It is challenging to explain supramental consciousness. Every aspect of human nature is conscious of its unity with the supreme here. There are two different types of movements involved in this trip from lower to higher consciousness: inward movement and upward movement. The upward movement raises the mind to the supramental level, which has the power to change the lower sections or the entirety of the being or nature, whereas the inward journey reveals the psychic (Manonmaniam Sundaranar University, n.d.). In short, Aurobindo's system is a thorough psychological framework that allows for the coexistence of both the modern and Indian perspectives. Comparative to other viewpoints, **integral psychology** actually provides a more comprehensive picture of human personality and psychological functioning.

One of the most prevalent interpretations of the Indian perspective on reality and existence is the **Advaita Vedanta System**, which has many characteristics in common with the majority of other schools. The self's nature and the nature of reality as a whole are seen by the Advaita Vedanta. It asserts that the self is a permanent entity that cannot be split up or destroyed. The death of the body does not kill the self. One achieves immortality by realizing the unchanging self that lies behind all changes. It is outside of senses, intuition, and mind. The self cannot be located or observed within physical bodies. Since it has no physical form, it exists everywhere, like space. Through the practice of yoga, which helps to restrain the five senses, concentrate the mind and settle the intellect, one can perceive self. As a result, core nature, which lies beneath all forms, is transcendental. Practising Advaita Vedanta theories and living life in the way guided by Advaita Vendanta is the core and essence of Hindu philosophy. Here we can find both the roots and the goals of all sciences and paradigms.

References

Ahuja, S. (2015). Ayurveda and modern psychology. *American International Journal of Research in Humanities, Arts and Social Sciences, 11*(3), 213–216.

Akhilananda, S. (1948). *Hindu psychology: Its meaning for the west*. Routledge.

Alexander, C. H. (1990). Growth of higher stages of consciousness: Maharishi Vedic psychology on human development. In C. H. Alexander & E. Langer (Eds.), *Higher stages of human development: Perspectives on adult growth*. Oxford University Press.

Alexander, C. N., & Bodeker, G. C. (1982). *Toward a theory and measurement of post conceptual stages of development*. Paper presented at the 90th annual meeting of the American Psychological Association.

Alexander, C. N., Boyer, R., & Alexander, V. (1987). Higher states of consciousness in the Vedic psychology of Maharishi Mahesh Yogi: A theoretical introduction and research review. *Modern Science and Vedic Science, 1*(1), 89–126.

Alexander, C. N., & Boyer, R. W. (1989). Seven states of consciousness. *Modern Science and Vedic Science, 2*(4), 325–371.

Alexander, V. K. (2005). Applications of Maharishi Vedic science to developmental psychology. *Journal of Social Behavior and Personality, 17*(1), 9–20.

American Psychiatric Association. (2013). *Diagnostic and statistical manual of mental disorders* (5th ed.). American Psychiatric Publishing.

Aron, A., Orme-Johnson, D., & Brubaker, P. (1981). The Transcendental Meditation program in the college curriculum: A 4-year longitudinal study of effects on cognitive and affective functioning. *College Student Journal, 15*(2), 140–146.

Arsh, P. (1999). *Atharvediya Mantra Vidya*. Gurukul Kangri Press.

Aurobindo, S. (1999). *The synthesis of Yoga* (5th ed.). Sri Aurobindo Ashram Trust.

Baer, R. A. (2003). Mindfulness training as a clinical intervention: A conceptual and empirical review. *Clinical Psychology, Science and Review, 10*, 125–143. https://doi.org/10.1093/clipsy.bpg015

Balaji Deekshitulu, P. V. (2019). Astrology and mental health. *International Journal of Philosophical Research, 1*(1), 1–4. https://escipub.com/Articles/IJOPR/IJPR-2019-06-2505.pdf

Basu, S. (2001). Integral psychotherapy: Personal encounters. In: M. Cornelissen (Ed.), *Consciousness and its transformation* (pp. 89–97). Sri Aurobindo International Centre of Education: Sri Aurobindo Ashram Pondicherry.

Behere, P. B. (2013). Ayurvedic concepts related to psychotherapy. *Indian Journal of Psychiatry, 55*(2), 310–314. PMC. http://www.ncbi.nlm.nih.gov/pmc/articles/PMC3705701/

Berg, A. L., Sandahl, C., & Bullington, J. (2010). Patients' perspective of change processes in affect-focused body psychotherapy for generalised anxiety disorder. *Body, Movement and Dance in Psychotherapy, 5*(2), 151–169. https://doi.org/10.1080/17432979.2010.494853

Bhatia, S. C., Madabushi, J., Kolli, V., Bhatia, S. K., & Madaan, V. (2013). The Bhagavad Gita and contemporary psychotherapies. *Indian Journal of Psychiatry, 55*(2), 315–321. https://doi.org/10.4103/0019-5545.105557

Bhawuk, D. P. S. (2011). *Spirituality and Indian Psychology: Lessons from the Bhagavad-Gita*. Springer.

Brisbon, N. M., & Lowery, G. A. (2011). Mindfulness and levels of stress: A comparison of beginner and advanced Hatha Yoga practitioners. *Journal of Religion and Health, 50*(4), 931–941. https://doi.org/10.1007/s10943-009-9305-3

Brown, R. P., & Gerbarg, P. L. (2009). Yoga breathing, meditation, and longevity. *Annals of the New York Academy of Sciences, 1172*, 54–62. https://doi.org/10.1111/j.1749-6632.2009.04394.x

Burton, R. (1964). *The Perfumed Garden of the Sheikh Nafzawi (Translated)*. Castle Books.

Burton, R., & Arbuthnot, F. F. (1984). *The Kamasutra of Vatsyayana (Translated)*. Putnam.

Caplan, M., Portillo, A., & Seely, L. (2013). Yoga psychotherapy: The integration of western psychological theory and ancient yogic wisdom. *The Journal of Transpersonal Psychology, 45*(2), 139–158.

Chakraborty, K., & Thakurata, R. G. (2013). Indian concepts on sexuality. *Indian Journal of Psychiatry, 55*, 250–255.

Chandra, B. V. (1978). *Ayurveda Mano Darshan, Pryoga Gata o Tattva Gata* (pp. 43–62). Haralal Bardhan.

Collins, J. H. (2008). *A to Z of palmistry, the essentials for reading hands*. JAICO.

Cornelissen, R. M. M., Misra, G., & Varma, S. (2014). Introduction to the second edition. In M. Cornelissen, G. Misra, & S. Varma (Eds.), *Foundations and applications of Indian Psychology* (2nd ed.) (pp. xi–xxv). Dorling Kindersley.

Dabas, P., & Singh, A. (2018). Bhagavad Gita teachings and positive psychology: Efficacy for semi-urban Indian students of NCR. *Cogent Psychology, 5*(1), 1467255. https://doi.org/10.1080/23311908.2018.1467255

Dalal, A. K. (n.d.). A journey back to the roots: Psychology in India. In M. Cornelisson, G. Misra, & S. Verma (Eds.), *Foundations of Indian psychology*. Pearson. https://www.ipi.org.in/texts/ajit/dalal-joureny-to-the-roots.pdf

Daniel, R. (2014). Ayurvedic psychology: Ancient wisdom meets modern science. *International Journal of Transpersonal Studies, 33*(1), 158–171.

Danielou, A. (1993). *The complete Kama Sutra: The first unabridged modern translation of the classic Indian text*. Inner Traditions.

Das, R. C. (1991). Standardization of the Gita inventory of personality. *Journal of Indian Psychology, 9*, 47–55.

Dasgupta, S. (1952). *History of Indian Philosophy* (Vol. II). Cambridge University Press.

Dash, B. (2008). *Caraka Samhita*. Chowkhamba Press.

David, R. (1978). *The birth of Indian psychology and its development in Buddhism*. Oriental Books Reprint Corporation.

Dhakad, M. K. (2018). Critical analysis of psychological concepts in the Bhagavad Gita. *International Journal of Science and Research, 7*(2), 471–476. https://www.ijsr.net/archive/v7i2/ART20179924.pdf

Dillbeck, M. C., & Alexander, C. N. (1989). Higher states of consciousness: Maharishi Mahesh Yogi's Vedic psychology of human development. *The Journal of Mind and Behavior, 10*(4), 307–334. http://www.jstor.org/stable/43853469.

Dutt, S. (2006). *India in a globalized world*. Manchester University Press.

Emerson, D., Sharma, R., Chaudhry, S., & Turner, J. (2009). Yoga therapy in practice: Trauma-sensitive yoga principles, practice, and research. *International Journal of Yoga Therapy, 19*, 123–128.

Fabrega, H. J. (2001). Mental health and illness in traditional India and China. *Cultural Psychiatry: International, 24*(3), 555–567.

Forbes, B. (2008). Using integrative yoga therapeutics in the treatment of comorbid anxiety and depression. *International Journal of Yoga Therapy, 18*, 87–95.

Fouw, H. D., & Svoboda, R. (2003). *Light on life: An introduction to the astrology of India*. Lotus Press.

Frawley, D. (1997). *Ayurveda and the mind: The healing of consciousness*. Lotus Press.

Frawley, D. (2011). *Ayurveda and the mind* (5th ed.). Lotus Press.

Frawley, D. (2012). Ayurveda and the mind: An overview. *American Institute of Vedic Studies*. https://vedanet.com/2012/06/13/ayurveda-and-the-mind-an-overview/

Frawley, D., & Halpern, M. (2006). *Ayurvedic psychology: Anxiety and depression*. California College of Ayurveda.

Frederick, T. T. (2021). Consciousness is primary: Science of consciousness for the 21st century. *International Journal of Psychological Studies, 13*(1), 1–11. https://doi.org/10.5539/ijps.v13n1p1/

Gilbert, P. (2014). Compassion-focused therapy: Preface and introduction for special section. *British Journal of Clinical Psychology, 53*(1), 1–5. https://doi.org/10.1111/bjc.12045

Gootjes, L., Franken, I. H. A., & Van Strien, J. W. (2011). Cognitive emotion regulation in yogic meditative practitioners: Sustained modulation of electrical brain potentials. *Journal of Psychophysiology, 25*(2), 87–94. https://doi.org/10.1027/0269-8803/a000043

Granath, J. (2006). Stress management: A randomized study of cognitive behavioural therapy and yoga. *Cognitive Behaviour Therapy, 35*(1), 3–10. https://doi.org/10.1080/16506070500401292

Green, M. B. (1986). Superstrings. *Scientific American, 255*(3), 48–60.

Haksar, A. N. D., & Favre, M. (2011). *Kama Sutra*. Penguin.

Halpern, M. (2010). *Principles of Ayurvedic medicine: Tenth edition*. California College of Ayurveda.

Harper, J. (2010). Teaching Yoga in urban elementary schools. *International Journal of Yoga Therapy, 1*(1), 99–109.

Harvard Health Publications. (2009). Yoga for anxiety and depression. *Harvard Mental Health Letter.* Retrieved July 26, 2022, from http://www.health.harvard.edu/newsletters/Harvard_Mental_Health_Letter/2009/April/Yoga-for-anxiety-and-depression

Hume, D. (1962). *The principal Upanishads.* Motilal Banarshidass.

Jevning, R., Wilson, A. F., & Davidson, J. M. (1978). Adrenocortical activity during meditation. *Hormones and Behavior, 10*, 525.

Jung, C.G. (1999). The development of the idea of collective unconscious and of archetypes. In A. Storr (Ed.), *The Essential Jung.* Fontana Press.

Karambelkar, V. W. (1959). *Civilization.* Nagpur University Press.

Karani, M. (2014). Understanding vernacular: Vastu shastra and Carl Jung's theories of psychology. *Journal of the International Society for the Study of Vernacular Settlements, 3*(1), 20–29.

Karatsoreos, I. N. (2014). Links between circadian rhythms and psychiatric disease. *Frontiers in Behavioral Neuroscience, 8*, 162. PMC. http://www.ncbi.nlm.nih.gov/pmc/articles/PMC4018537/

Katakkar, M. (1992). *Encyclopedia of Palm and Palm Reading.* UBSPD.

Kinser, P. A., Bourguignon, C., Whaley, D., Hauenstein, E., & Taylor, A. G. (2013). Feasibility, acceptability, and effects of gentle hatha yoga for women with major depression: Findings from a randomized controlled mixed-methods study. *Archives of Psychiatric Nursing, 27*(3), 137–147. https://doi.org/10.1016/j.apnu.2013.01.003

Kumar, C. N. R., Chandra, P. G., & Narayana, R. (2011). Future pathway to biometrics. *International Journal of Biometrics and Bioinformatics, 5*(3), 180–190.

Kumar, M., & Chaudhari, N. (2016). Concept of psychology and the mind in Ayurveda. *International Ayurvedic Medical Journal, 4*(3), 540–547.

Labbe-Watson, J. (2020). *Ayurvedic and Bionian theories of thinking: Mental digestion and the truth instinct* [Ph.D. Dissertation]. Antioch University, New England. https://aura.antioch.edu/etds/596

Lad, V. (1995). An introduction to Ayurveda. *Alternative Therapies in Health and Medicine, 1*(3), 57–63.

Lad, V. (2002). *Textbook of Ayurveda: Fundamental Principles of Ayurveda* (Vol. 1). The Ayurvedic Press.

Lad, V. (2006). *Textbook of Ayurveda: A complete guide to clinical assessment* (1st ed.). The Ayurvedic Press.

Lalande, L., Bambling, M., King, R., & Lowe, R. (2012). Breathwork: An additional treatment option for depression and anxiety. *Journal of Contemporary Psychotherapy, 42*(2), 113–119. http://search.proquest.com/docview/941017476?accountid525260

Leahy, R. L. (1996). *Cognitive therapy: Basic principles and applications.* Jason Aronson Publishing Co.

Logan, A. C., & Felice, N. J. (2014). Nutritional psychiatry research: An emerging discipline and its intersection with global urbanization, environmental challenges and the evolutionary mismatch. *Journal of Physiological Anthropology, 33*(1), 22. PMC. http://www.ncbi.nlm.nih.gov/pmc/articles/PMC4131231/

Lopez, G. (2011). Why verbal psychotherapy is not enough to treat post-traumatic stress disorder: A biosystemic approach to stress debriefing. *Body, Movement and Dance in Psychotherapy, 6*(2), 129–143. https://doi.org/10.1080/17432979.2011.583060

Maharishi Mahesh Yogi. (1963). *Science of being and the art of living.* Signet.

Maharishi Mahesh Yogi. (1969). *On the Bhagavad-Gita: A new translation and commentary.* Penguin.

Maharishi Mahesh Yogi. (1972). *Science of creative intelligence: Knowledge and experience.* MIU Press.

Maharishi Mahesh Yogi. (1977). *Creating an ideal society.* MERU Press.

Maharishi Mahesh Yogi. (1986). *Life supported by natural law.* Age of Enlightenment Press.

Maharishi Mahesh Yogi. (1994). *Maharishi Vedic University: Introduction*. Maharishi Vedic University Press.

Maharishi Mahesh Yogi. (1997). *Celebrating perfection in education*. Maharishi Vedic University Press.

Manickam, L. S. S. (2005). Development of a personality tool based on Upanishadic concepts: Conceptual and methodological issues. In K. R. Rao & S. B. Marwaha (Eds.), *Towards a spiritual psychology: Essays in Indian psychology* (1st ed.). SAMVAD India Foundation.

Manonmaniam Sundaranar University. (n.d.). *Indigenous psychology*. Directorate of Distance and Continuing Education, Tirunelveli, Tamil Nadu, India. Retrieved August 07, 2022, from https://www.msuniv.ac.in/Download/Pdf/9d2778d7aa7e41d

Mathew, V. G. (1994). *IAS Inventory and Manual*. Deparment of Psychology, University of Kerala.

Mathew, V. G. (2001) Models of consciousness and its transformation. In M. Cornelissen (Ed.), *Consciousness and its transformation* (pp. 189–198). Sri Aurobindo International Center of Education: Sri Aurobindo Ashram Pondicherry.

Mathew, V. G. (n.d.). *A short history of Indian psychology*. Retrieved July 24, 2022, from https://web.archive.org/web/20150130013217/http://www.psychology4all.com/historyi.htm

Matthijs, C. (2002). Pondicherry manifesto of Indian psychology. *Psychological Studies, 47*(1–3), 168–169.

McKeithen, B. (n.d.). Indian psychology. *History of Psychology in the East*. Retrieved July 27, 2022, from https://psychologyoftheeast.umwblogs.org/indian-psychology/

Mehling, W. E., Wrubel, J., Daubenmier, J. J., Price, C. J., Kerr, C. E., Silow, T., Gopisetty, V., & Stewart, A. L. (2011). Body awareness: A phenomenological inquiry into the common ground of mind-body therapies. *Philosophy, Ethics, and Humanities in Medicine, 6*(1), 1–12. https://doi.org/10.1186/1747-5341-6-6

Menon, B. (2016). Comprehensive analysis of personality—An Ayurvedic perspective. *International Journal of Indian Psychology, 3*(3), 99–111. DIP: 18.01.108/20160303/99–111.

Miller, R. C. (1994). The breath of life: Through the practice of pranayama, the regulation of the breath, we can learn to bring forth and direct the spiritual energy that underlies all life. *Yoga Journal, 116*, 82.

Misra, G. (2011). *Handbook of psychology in India*. Oxford University Press.

Mohan, V., & Sandhu, S. (1986). Development of a scale to measure sattvic, rajasic and tamasic guna. *Journal of Indian Academy of Applied Psychology, 12*, 46–52.

Moore, S. (2018). *The three doshas and the mind in Ayurveda*. https://nayaAyurveda.com/taxonomy/term/229

Mukherjee, R. (2007). Concept of personality type in West and in Ayurveda. *Indian Journal of Traditional Knowledge, 6*(3), 432–438.

Nichter, M. (2008). Coming to our senses: Appreciating the sensorial in medical anthropology. *Transcultural Psychiatry, 45*(2), 163–197. https://doi.org/10.1177/1363461508089764

Obeyesekere, G. (1977). The theory and practice of psychological medicine in the Ayurvedic tradition. *Culture, Medicine and Psychiatry, 2*(1), 155–181. https://doi.org/10.1007/BF00114848

Orme-Johnson, D. W. (2000). An overview of Charles Alexander's contribution to psychology: Developing higher states of consciousness in the individual and the society. *Journal of Adult Development, 7*(4), 199–215.

Panda, M. (2019). Historical lapses and contemporary perspective in biometrics. *International Journal of Jyotish Research, 4*(2), 1–3.

Patwardhan, B., Joshi, K., & Chopra, A. (2005). Classification of human population based on HLA gene polymorphism and the concept of *prakriti* in Ayurveda. *Journal of Alternative and Complementary Medicine, 11*(2), 349–353. https://doi.org/10.1089/acm.2005.11.349

Piaget, J., & Inhelder, B. (1969). *The psychology of the child*. Basic Books.

Prasad, M. N. (1995). *The Kena Upanishad*. D. K. Printworld.

Prasad, S. (2012). Human face architecture and structure of eyes for prediction of mental state of individual. *International Journal of Scientific and Research Publications, 2*(4), 20–29.

Prasuna, V. V. L., Sharma, B. K., & Narayana, A. (2014). Comparative study of personality with Ayurvedic prakriti. *International Journal of Ayur Pharma Research, 2*(1), 124–136.

Price, C. (2005). Body-oriented therapy in recovery from child sexual abuse: An efficacy study. *Alternative Therapies in Health and Medicine, 11*(5), 46–57.

Privitera, C. M., & Stark, L. W. (2000). Algorithms for defining visual regions of interest: Comparison with eye fixations. *IEEE Transactions on Pattern Analysis and Machine Intelligence, 22*(9), 970–982.

Rao, K. R. (2008). Prologue: Introducing Indian psychology. In K. R. Rao, A. C. Paranjpe, & A. K. Dalal (Eds.), *Handbook of Indian psychology* (pp. 1–18). Cambridge University Press India.

Rao, K. R., & Paranjpe, A. C. (2016). *Psychology in the Indian Tradition.* Springer. https://doi.org/10.1007/978-81-322-2440-2

Rao, P. S. (2007). *Manas: Psychiatry of Ayurveda.* Chowkhamba Prakashan.

Rao, S. (1997). Salvation: A Hindu perspective. *World Faiths Encounter, 18*, 11–20.

Ravi, K. V., Chiplunkar, S., & Shetty, S. K. (2013). A pilot study on design and validation of Manasika Prakriti questionnaire. *Journal of Ayurveda and Holistic Medicine, 1*(2), 15–25.

Reddy, G. N. N., Ramut, M. G., & Venkataram, B. S. (1987). Concept of *manas* (psyche) in Ayurveda. *NIMHANS Journal, 5*(2), 125–131.

Rhoda, D. (2014). Ayurvedic psychology: Ancient wisdom meets modern science. *International Journal of Transpersonal Studies, 33*(1), 158–171. https://doi.org/10.24972/ijts.2014.33.1.158

Roger, B. (2013). Samkhya cosmogeny in asana. Retrieved from https://yogastlouis.us/samkhyacosmogeny-in-asana/#_ftn42

Salagame, K. K. K. (1988). States of consciousness: Perspectives from modern psychology. In M. A. S. Rajan (Ed.), *Consciousness: Proceedings of the workshop.* The Academy of Sanskrit Research.

Salagame, K. K. K. (2002). *Psychology of meditation: A contextual approach.* Concept Publishing Co.

Salagame, K. K. K. (2010a). Psychology of yoga and yoga psychology. In *Yoga—The light of microuniverse* (conference proceedings). Yoga Federation of Serbia.

Salagame, K. K. K. (2010b, June 23–27). Need for the distinction between transpersonal and transcendental. *Consciousness Revolution.* In *17th International Transpersonal Conference.*

Salagame, K. K. K. (2013). Indian psychology. In K. D. Keith (Ed.), *The encyclopedia of cross-cultural psychology* (1st ed.). Wiley. https://onlinelibrary.wiley.com/doi/epdf/10.1002/9781118339893.wbeccp283

Santon, M. Y. (2008). *How to read* (Vol. 2). Ajay Book Publishing.

Sara, T., Härenstam, A., & Hagberg, M. (2011). Mobile phone use and stress, sleepdisturbances, and symptoms of depression among young adults—A prospective cohort study. *BMC Public Health 11* 66. PMC. http://www.ncbi.nlm.nih.gov/pmc/articles/PMC3042390/

Sengupta, K. D., & Sengupta, K. U. (1916). *Astanga Hrdaya-Srimad Vagbhatta Birachita.* Reference retrieved from *Indian Journal of Traditional Knowledge, 6*(3), July 2007, pp. 432–438. http://14.139.47.15/bitstream/123456789/975/1/IJTK%206%283%29%20%282007%29%20432-438.pdf

Serber, E. (2000). Stress management through yoga. *International Journal of Yoga Therapy, 10*, 11–16.

Sharma, N. (2014a). Cognitive behaviour therapy in perspective of the Bhagwat Gita. *International Journal of Humanities and Social Science Invention, 3*(1), 2319–7722.

Sharma, N. (2014b). The Bhagwat Gita as a complimentary tool to cognitive behavioral therapy. *International Journal of Applied Psychology, 4*(2), 45–49. https://doi.org/10.5923/j.ijap.20140402.01

Sharma, P. V. (1981). *Caraka Samhita* (pp. 434–439). Chowkhamba Prakashan.

Sharma, R. K., & Dash, V. B. (1977). *Caraka Samhita Vol II* (pp. 404–413). Chowkhamba Prakashan.

Shashtri, K. (1951). *Further lights: The vedas and tantra.* Sri Aurobindo Ashram Press.

Shukla, V., & Tripathi, R. (2011). *Vaidyamanorama Sutra-Sthan, Hindi commentary.* Charak Samhita. Chaukhambha Sanskrit Pratisthan.

Shilpa, S., & Murthy, C. G. V. (2011). Understanding personality from Ayurvedic perspective for psychological assessment: A case. *AYU Journal, 32*(1), 12–19. https://doi.org/10.4103/0974-8520.85716

Singer, M., & Le Vine, R. A. (2001). Culture and personality studies. *Journal of Personality, 69*(6), 803–818.

Singh, H. G. (1977). *Psychotherapy in India.* H.P.

Singh, R. H. (2010). Exploring larger evidence-base for contemporary Ayurveda. *International Journal of Ayurvedic Research, 1*(1), 65–66. https://doi.org/10.4103/0974-7788.64394

Sinha, J. (1933). *Indian Psychology* (Vols. 1 and 2). Kegan Paul.

Spinazzola, J., Rhodes, A. M., Emerson, D., Earle, E., & Monroe, K. (2011). Application of yoga in residential treatment of traumatized youth. *Journal of the American Psychiatric Nurses Association, 17*(6), 431–444. https://doi.org/10.1177/1078390311418359

Steckler, L., & Young, C. (2009). Depression and body psychotherapy. *International Journal of Psychotherapy, 13*(2), 32–41.

Suchitra, S. P., Gangadhar, B. N., Nagarathna, R., & Nagendra, H. R. (2010). Measuring the tridosha symptoms of unmada (psychosis): A preliminary study. *Journal of Alternative and Complementary Medicine, 16*(4), 457–462. https://doi.org/10.1089/acm.2009.0296

Sundaravadivelu, S. (2013). Study of cosmic radiation and human health. *International Journal of Innovative Research in Computer and Communication Engineering, 1*(7), 1379.

Sundaravadivelu, S. (2014). Study of cosmic intelligence and human health. *International Journal of Innovative Research in Computer and Communication Engineering, 2*(5), 4325.

Suneeta, S., & Shrikrishna, C. (2009). Triguna personality theory: Classical representation and modern research. *Journal of Indian Psychology, 27* (1 and 2), 35–46.

Svoboda, R. E. (2004). *Ayurveda: Life, health, and longevity.* The Ayurvedic Press.

Svoboda, R. E. (1999). *Your Ayurvedic constitution: Prakruti.* Lotus Press.

Tatavarthy, B. B. R. V. (2007). Integrated concept of medical astrology and Ayurveda. *The Journal of Research and Education in Indian Medicine.* https://www.researchgate.net/publication/283070178_INTEGRATED_CONCEPT_OF_MEDICAL_ASTROLOGY_AND_AYURVEDA

Teja, J. S. (1971). Proposed classification of other psychoses for use in India. *Indian Journal of Psychiatry, 13*, 7–13.

Tirtha, S. S. (1998). *The Ayurvedic encyclopedia: Natural secrets to healing, prevention, and longevity.* Ayurveda Holistic Center Press.

Tjoa, A. (1975). Meditation, neuroticism and intelligence: A follow up. *Gedrag: Tijdschrift Voor Psychologie (Behavior: Journal of Psychology), 3,* 167–182.

Travis, F. (2015). *How meditation heals: The brain and higher states of consciousness.* Lowman and Littlefield.

Travis, F. (2018). Long term changes in experienced yoga practitioners: Growth of higher states of consciousness in TM subjects. *IGI Global.* https://doi.org/10.4018/978-1-5225-2788-6.ch003

Tripathi, B. (2001). *Charak Samhita, Vaidya–Chandrika (Sharir Sthan), Hindi Vyakhya—Part II.* Chaukhambha Surbharati Prakashan.

Upadhyaya, S. C. (1965). *Kama Sutra of Vatsyayana complete translation from the original Sanskrit.* DB Taraporevala.

Van, D. K. (2006). Clinical implications of neuroscience research in PTSD. *Annals of the New York Academy of Sciences, 1071*, 277–293.

Van Loon, G. (ed.) (2002). *Charaka Samhita: Handbook on Ayurveda* (Vol. 2). Chaukhambha Orientalia.

Venkobarao, A. (2002). Mind in Ayurveda. *Indian Journal of Psychiatry, 44*(3), 201–211.

Visagratna, K. L. (1981). *Sushruta Samhita* (Vol. II) (pp. 154–158). Chowkhamba Sanskrit Series.

Walia, M., & Singh, H. (2018). Ayurveda and psychology. *World Journal of Pharmaceutical Research, 7*(2), 224–231.

Wallace, R. K. (1986). *The Maharishi technology of the unified field: The neurophysiology of enlightenment.* MIU Press.

Weintraub, A. (2004). *Yoga for depression.* Broadway Books.

Welch, C. (2005). *Secrets of the mind: The 10 channels revealed*. Big Shakti Press.
Wendy, D. (2003). The Kamasutra: It isn't all about sex. *The Kenyon Review. New Series, 25*(1), 18–37.
Wendy, D. (2016). *Redeeming the Kamasutra*. Oxford University Press.
Wendy, D., & Sudhir, K. (2002). *Kamasutra*. Oxford World's Classics: Oxford University Press.
Wig, N. N., & Singh, G. (1967). A proposed classification of psychiatric disorders for use in India. *Indian Journal of Psychiatry, 8*, 157–171.
Wolf, D. B. (1996). A psychometric analysis of the three gunas. *Journal of Indian Psychology, 16*, 26–43.
Wolf, D. B. (1999). A psychometric analysis of the three gunas. *Psychological Reports, 84*(13), 79–90.